Bundle 2 in 1: Emotional Healthy Spirituality & Emotional Agility Guidebook

How to Manage Self-Esteem, Stop Negative Thinking & Anxiety and Create Emotional intelligence, Emotional Design & Detox

Caryl R. Breton

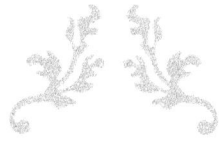

EMOTIONAL DESIGN & EMOTIONAL AGILITY TO MANAGE SELF-ESTEEM PILLARS:

Social Emotional Learning Book: How to Win Solitude and Loneliness, Create Empathy & Emotional intelligence, and Your Own Depression Cure

Contents

11 pm   2

Penn Mar Ave, California.   2

Chapter 1: "I'm like you even if you don't know it."   19

Chapter 2: When the nights are blue and there's no meaning to it   37

Chapter 3: The Global Crisis of Mental Health   55

Chapter 4: The advent of empathy and emotional intelligence in our lives   66

Chapter 5: Emotional intelligence in design and marketing   84

Chapter 6: The Black Dog   96

11 pm

Penn Mar Ave, California.

Sometimes you break. It is not only bodies that are vulnerable to blows. Life sometimes mistreats you. And it doesn't depend on what you do, how much you put in on your part. Resilience is also finite. Then you come undone. Although, of course, as with objects, sometimes you crack inside, even if the eye does not see it.

And then, at another point and for hardly significant reasons, the cracks in your being say that they no longer support more weight. When it starts, it may be nothing more than an intense feeling of discomfort. A kind of omnipresent restlessness that accompanies you wherever you go and stays with you, whatever you do.

You feel that something is wrong, although you cannot identify it. It is a state of restlessness that deprives you of calm. Unhappiness does not go away, and that clouds your pleasant moments. It is that unbearable feeling of wanting everything to end, for the present to disappear, for the moment to cease to be eternal. It is displeasure that gnaws at your insides. You stop sleeping.

Of all its manifestations, this, perhaps, is the cruelest because you stop dreaming. At least before you ran away from yourself at night. There is no more peace or oasis possible. You cannot disconnect from your thoughts; you do not escape discomfort.

Not even exhaustion breaks you as a refuge from that restlessness that burns you. At first, you stop enjoying yourself. Nothing satisfies you; everything irritates you. But it doesn't stop there. I don't know how to explain how it works, nor am I clear why it happens, but it is infallible: spiritual pain builds a physical shell for you. Not as a metaphor.

The surface of the skin dies. When you realize it, you already have the body of a zombie. You look at the ground and think: "Where did all that blood come from? What happened?". And then you discover that you have a glass nailed to the sole of your foot, you don't know for how long.

You remove it, and it doesn't hurt. You cook, you burn with oil, you blister, but you only know it because you see it. Touch does not respond. And the physical numbness seems proportional to the depth of the well. The deeper you are, the less you feel. The more it tears you apart from the inside, the more you disconnect from the outside. The deeper you are, the less you feel!

And with the ability to feel, your energies go away. Depression is a deficit of life, a void of being. And this lack, when it becomes present, empties everything. Because depression also has its peak, the point where existence breaks down.

At that moment, what we call identity becomes an empty facade, a farce. And I don't mean here that you are experiencing an identity crisis like the one that usually occurs in adolescence. It is not an evolution. It is dissolution.

You continue because you have built yourself an automatic pilot. Whether we know it or not, we have many automatisms, habits, even complex cognitive resources that continue to function on their own. But existing becomes unbearable.

How do you explain who has not been through something like that you want to end your life? Living is an instinct; they tell you. But so is avoiding suffering. Because putting a stop to pain is what moves you to do it. Imagine an agony that does not stop, that becomes unbearable, and to which you do not see the end. That is an episode of major depression. Once you fall beyond the edge of the abyss, down the ravine, you live like a doomed Prometheus. Perpetual suffering from which you can only escape by killing yourself.

Depression hurts. And it's not a metaphor. Suffering is not an abstraction. It's bad. You feel it in your chest, in your head, in your gut. That omnipresent discomfort and the feeling that it will always be this way. It is no coincidence that the two groups with the highest risk of suicide, attempted or completed, are major depression and those who live with chronic (physical) pain. Continual suffering is unsustainable.

Of course, major depression can come through. That is why we talk about episodes. Now at that moment, you don't know it, you don't believe it, you can't even conceive it. When you are inside, there is no end to suffering.

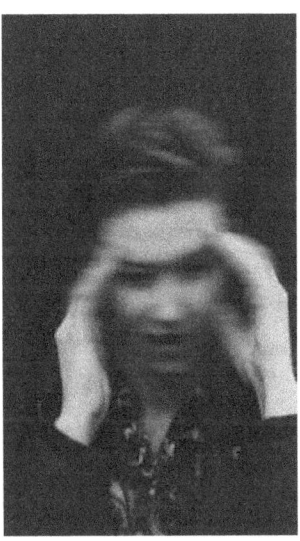

Perhaps when you recover, you can proudly say, "I survived myself." But at that moment, in full depression, it is unthinkable. You do not find motives or strength to bear so much suffering. No one can convince you that the blows will stop hurting in the middle of a beating. You just want them to end. Already. This is how a suicide attempt comes along.

How can it happen that you feel bad, feel the suffering, become aware that you are undone, and do not ask for help? Now, looking back, it's easy to explain. It is a stigma, and it is machismo. But when it is happening, you do not even suspect that your prejudices can drag you down the ravine, that they are a source of suffering, and affect your health.

Understanding why it happens is simple: we are not impervious to social prejudice. We look at ourselves in the mirror of the gaze of others. And if the social imaginary teaches us that receiving a mental health diagnosis, taking psychiatric drugs, or even worse, going through a psychiatric hospital stay is something for crazy people or emotionally weak people, it is clear that you are not "that."

You are not looking for help because you are scared to be diagnosed. Prejudice is a serious health problem. Because of it, you arrive at the services when you are already in a crisis, you have more difficulties recovering, and you may end up much worse in your process.

And concerning depression, precisely, gender-dependent differences can be explained in terms of stereotypes of sexual roles. Although there is a greater propensity to label women with depression, men are usually diagnosed when we have more severe symptoms. I was no exception. The fear of the labor and social consequences that the label could bring me was also a strong reason not to ask for help.

Now, empowered and overcome with fear and shame, I can say, as I always do, that it should come as no surprise that I am an individual living with a diagnosis of severe mental disorder; that no person, regardless of their training, trade or profession is free from the possibility of experiencing a mental health problem.

Education can bring us many things, but it does not immunize against suffering. Now, of course, looking back, I can position myself from the security of a life that also continues professionally. Back then, this security was inconceivable. Returning to the world, once broken and labeled, is scary.

Back home, it took me more than two months to get out of a room. Beyond the weight of the symptoms and the over-medication, there was a lot of fear of what awaited me outside in this confinement.

Only in a space that enables and promotes being responsible for oneself and one's community is it possible to abandon the sick person's role and become empowered. Psychoeducation geared towards taking your medication is empowering; learning to iron is empowering; painting mandalas, taking a guided tour of the zoo, listening to a talk about empowerment, everything empowers. Of course, always, always, these are activities offered by professionals for users. Power, of course, comes from above.

Now, in concrete terms, what is empowerment? How do you get it? According to Rappaport's definition: "Empowerment is a process, the mechanism by which people, organizations and communities acquire dominion over their lives."

It is clear, therefore, that painting mandalas do not grant control over our existence. Nor is learning basic skills for personal autonomy empowering. Even the simple act of making decisions does not have this effect.

If that were the case, every time they ask us if we want chicken or meat dürum, they would be empowering us, choosing the movie for the next Netflix Party or the site for the next excursion are not elections that meet the conditions to empower people.

Something more is needed. In this regard, by specifically defining the elements of empowerment in mental health, Judi Chamberlin stressed that empowerment does not only have decision-making power but that these decisions should make it possible to effect changes in one's life and the community. The need for self-management, without labels or people acting as professionals, is precisely to dismantle the reciprocal game that perpetuates the sick role.

The path of activism looks different. It is no longer about breaking prejudices and showing that the first person's associative movement is possible, effective, and transformative. Towards the same horizon, along parallel paths, we have been growing different people and entities. Today it is not all desert or hostile land.

It is no longer just a matter of building a refuge in which to find ourselves, remake ourselves, and recover. Shame has become vindication. It is no longer a personal search. In that sense, I think I have found all that I had lost.

Helen

"I could expect it from someone else, but not from you," I replied when she told me.

I had said it with good intentions, claiming her strength and her profession, but anxiety does not work like that. It can affect anyone, just like so many other diseases.

The following account shares the story of my sister, Helen, and her long battle with anxiety. I bring her story as an overarching reference to my book's central idea and the ever-forgotten aspect of mental health, its wild spontaneity, and its labyrinth.

I am a psychologist, and I suffer from anxiety, yes.

On September 11 of last year, I suffered my first panic attack. At the time, it was not clear to me what was happening to me. Yes, now it is. But let us start at the beginning. It was a normal day. It was no worse than other days.

What's more, it was one of the best moments of that year – he had asked me out just two days ago!! – everything was as good as it could be. However, that morning, while I was working, I had coffee – the second in the morning – like many other days.

When I finished the cup, I began to feel dizzy, breathing difficulties, chest tightness, tachycardia, sweaty hands, fear of fainting, having a stroke, a heart attack. Terror. Fear of dying. All of this accompanied by the fear of fainting in public, ultimately losing control of myself and my body. Coffee wasn't the culprit, of course.

Think of six people in your environment. Keep them in your memory. Now consider that, according to the available estimates, one of those six people will suffer at some point in their life an anxiety disorder:

- *Panic attacks*
- *Agoraphobia*
- *Specific phobias*
- *Social phobia*
- *Generalized anxiety disorder*
- *Post-traumatic stress disorder*
- *Acute stress disorder*

- *Obsessive-compulsive disorder*
- *Unspecified anxiety disorder*

With this personal account, I do not intend to give keys to overcome a disorder of this type, nor will I offer magic recipes. My claim is more modest: to help normalize a disorder that can affect us all, either directly or close people. And within that 'everyone,' of course, mental health professionals are not excluded.

And yes, I am a psychologist, and I have suffered (suffer) from an anxiety disorder. In principle, my training should not be relevant in this, but perhaps it is surprising that one of the phrases that I have heard the most in recent months has been, "do you have anxiety being a psychologist?" You know who asked that one.

When I was in the mood to answer, my answer was, "to think that a psychologist cannot suffer from some kind of mental health problem is like thinking that a doctor cannot catch a cold." Neither psychologists nor any other professional is exempt from suffering health problems. In my case, I discovered that I did not seem to have more tools than the common man to cope with this disorder.

A few years ago, a very close friend began to suffer from anxiety problems. I allowed myself the luxury of giving him some advice – to see a mental health professional, do relaxation techniques, etc. – but when it was my turn, I could not apply any of that advice. And it is that, as they say, "in the house of a blacksmith, a wooden knife."

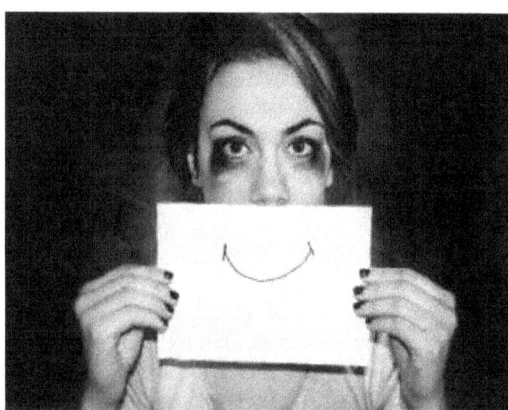

I would be lying if I said that the first panic attack was the beginning of my anxiety problems, just as it was not the worst part of this process. It all started about two years ago.

At first, the anxiety presented with mild symptoms: isolated nights and distant in time. The physical symptoms were difficulty falling asleep, the sensation of having a stiff jaw and difficulty swallowing.

However, other types of symptoms distressed me more: I felt dizzy, and I was afraid to fall asleep, in case I had some kind of attack, a stroke, a stroke, and I died during the night without knowing it. I was afraid of falling asleep and never waking up again. Anguish and fear kept me awake until I fell asleep from sheer exhaustion.

It was not difficult for me to realize that they were symptoms of anxiety. No, I knew it very soon, probably due to my training, but that did not make me give it the importance it deserved. On the one hand, I did not want to accept that it was possible that I had a problem of this type and, on the other, I believed that it was something temporary and I could control it myself. That was my first mistake.

This situation lasted for months: when I was out of work and had difficulty finding it, another time when I suffered from emotional disappointment, etc. My discomfort, sleepless nights, and dizziness that I did not know where they came from just after consuming exciting things (coffee, soda, etc.) worsened slightly with the diagnosis and progress of the terminal illness of one of the most important people of my life – my late best friend, Rory.

I have always been a very sensitive person; my family and friends laugh at me because I cry about everything. However, throughout his illness and after his death, I was not able to cry. I was completely blank and was unable to explain my emotions or accept what had happened.

Finding the cause of what happens to us is not easy. There is not a single one, and we do not have a way to find it, but I think this situation was the last straw. My fear of dying myself, or one of the people I love, increased, and appeared at the most unexpected moments and in the most varied way.

When I least expected it, fear attacked me and left me frozen and paralyzed. Even today, I don't know how to explain the feeling of cold in my stomach, as if all the blood was suddenly lost. I remember a time when I was walking down the street in high heels. I began to think that I might trip, not keep my balance, fall, and smash my head against the ground. It was not just the thought that it might happen, but real fear, which paralyzed me,

Some everyday situations, such as taking the subway, began to worry me about the risk of having an accident. I stopped reading newspapers or watching the news because every news about accidents or unexpected deaths distressed me thinking that it could happen to me too. These thoughts were presented with intense fear, sweaty hands, and some tachycardia. Also, around that time, I began to experience more and more difficulty sleeping.

In any case, those moments were brief. When I was distracted, I forgot them, so, although it worried me enough to discuss the situation with my family, I did not seek professional help either. I just took herbal remedies to try to sleep better and waited for it to go away on its own.

Second – and more serious – mistake.

That situation continued for a little over a month. After that, I went through a brief period in which I felt good, could sleep easily, and was not plagued by catastrophic thoughts. The period was very short, but I trusted myself, and I assumed that whatever was happening to me had already been solved and that, although I had come to consider it, I no longer needed professional help.

A few weeks later, I had my first panic attack.

As I write it, I wonder how I could not realize how serious the situation was and how much help I needed, but I was not, and being a psychologist did not facilitate it.

The same day of the first panic attack, moved by intense fear and uncontrollable anguish that I felt, I located a psychologist with training that convinced me and requested an appointment three days later.

Suffering from this situation and being overwhelmed made me understand that I needed help and could not control it alone. The fear of never getting over the situation by myself was what finally moved me. I didn't want to; I couldn't go through something like that again.

In addition to seeking psychological help, I went to my family doctor, referred from the emergency department, where I ended up after the first attack, where they used Lorazepam to control my attack. She proposed a drug treatment to me that, at first, I did not want to follow.

Two days after the first panic attack, I suffered the second while at home. Despite knowing what was happening to me and that it had happened to me before without major consequences, I could not handle it, and, again, I had to resort to Lorazepam since fear overwhelmed me. I still did not have the necessary tools to cope without drug help.

The worst was not the panic attacks, but the general state I found myself in each day after that second attack. I was constantly dizzy like it was on a boat, or the ground was completely uneven. I was distracted, tired, unable to pay attention, constantly aware of my condition, scared of having another attack. Fear did not give up. Fear and anguish.

I wasn't able to pay attention to the people around me. I went out with my friends or my family members, and I could not follow their conversations because discomfort and fear barely let me out of myself. I have forgotten the entire conversations and situations of those months.

And it's not that I didn't exactly remember the conversations, but they did ring a bell, but I don't remember that they happened at all. I have forgotten to have seen movies, have listened to songs, etc., totally completely. For months, I have been looking at myself for a dark part that haunted me.

And inside me, the recurring thoughts. They attacked me, and I was not able to control them. All related to death or accidents, with when and how I was going to die, with which all my relatives and loved ones would one day be gone, and I did not know when would be the last time I would see them.

Imagine the anguish that seeing your loved ones triggers the thought of whether that's the last time you'll see them. I got to the point where I passed people on the street, and I only thought about the years that those people had lived. I calculated how old they should be, and I thought that I was capable too if they had reached that age.

I thought over and over about the moment when it was time to die. I was afraid of getting old because I was approaching death. I wondered what it would be like if I would be afraid, or if I was older, I would no longer be. We all know that one day the people we love, and we will no longer be there, but we live day by day without thinking about it. However, for me, it was as if what I had always known that someone was there suddenly was lighting it up with a very powerful spotlight, and it was no longer able to look at anything else. The truth is that I feared that I would never be able to recover or fall into a depression.

During the first weeks, I have already mentioned it, I preferred not to take too much Lorazepam even though my doctor had recommended it to me. Professionally, I have always defended the combination of psychotherapy and controlled use of medication. Still, when it was my turn, I fell into the same prejudices as other people, and I was afraid of getting hooked, becoming tolerant, and needing more and more, etc. I tried treating myself only with psychotherapy, but most nights, I needed a sock or a pill to get to sleep.

The nights were, without a doubt, the worst time. I would arrive at nine o'clock at night with very high tension, I was shaking uncontrollably, and I was short of breath. It was like being terrified without interruption.

Once, on vacation with my partner, I found myself in the car shaking with fear, without him being able to do anything to comfort me, and nothing had happened. Anxiety and a feeling of loss of control go hand in hand. Fear gripped me, prevented me from eating, made me shiver as if I were freezing to death. Think of the most intense fear you have ever felt and imagine that it lasts for hours or even days.

Finally, I accepted the advice of my GP, whom I thank for her good work since from the first moment she treated me with respect, seriousness, and concern, and I began to take some medication – always under medical supervision and indication – at midafternoon to reach the calmer night.

Stopping feeling that intense and constant fear, thanks to the medication, helped me relax and take advantage of the therapy much more and better since I could finally begin to concentrate.

As for psychotherapy, it was very intense and deep work. It started by realizing that the anxiety did not come on suddenly but was due to my behavior patterns, stress management, coping with problems, lack of self-esteem, etc. And that not everything was limited to recent situations, but a whole history of the need for control, lack of assertiveness, low self-esteem, and problems of confidence in my abilities.

They were due to a catastrophic personality very focused on everything that could go wrong. Recent stressful situations have only pushed me to the limit.

The personal work of self-knowledge and change that I had to carry out during the time that the therapy lasted was not easy, nor was it free of pain, but I felt accompanied by my psychologist, by my family members, and by my friends, who from the first moment they knew what was happening to me.

I had to be very constant and put all my willpower into making an effort to take advantage of the therapy, carry out the proposals that my psychologist made me, and not give up even if it took time to see results.

Also, talking about my situation with my loved ones was very helpful as I discovered how many people had been through it, even within my closest family, without my knowing it. The testimony and support of others who had traveled a path similar to mine was helpful.

Almost a year has passed, and my anxiety has not disappeared or the personal work that I have to do every day has finished, but it no longer dominates me, it does not keep me sleepless every night, and it does not condition me.

Every day is an effort to keep changing and improving my behavior patterns and the negative thoughts that come upon me, but now I have the necessary tools and the motivation to do so, and I know that if I need to, I can go to my psychologist again. I have not completely changed my old habits, but now I am aware of what I was doing and doing to myself, and that helps me to be able to stop and look for different options. Therapy and personal work have made me aware of multiple avoidant attitudes and behaviors that I was carrying out without even realizing it.

As I said initially, no one is free from suffering from any type of illness, regardless of their profession, but anxiety disorders can be improved and managed with professional help. In my case, the help of psychotherapy and medication was necessary.

Each one should look for the option that best suits their needs but always seek professional help. It can be controlled; you can not only regain your normal life but improve it. But you cannot and do not have to do it alone. It does not matter if you are a psychologist, housewife, or astronaut.

We need help, and we must seek it both in our primary care medical center, where your family doctor will assess whether to treat you or refer you to the psychiatrist, as well as in a psychologist specialized in anxiety disorders.

Why I decided to write this book?

For most of my life, two mysteries hung over me. I didn't understand them, and if I'm honest, I was scared to investigate them. The first mystery is that I am in my 30s, and throughout my life, depression and anxiety have increased throughout the Western world.

I wanted to understand: why is this happening to us? Why is it so hard for so many more of us to get through the day?

And I wanted to understand this for a more personal mystery. When I was a teenager, I went to my doctor, and I remember telling him that I felt the pain was escaping me. I couldn't control it; I was quite ashamed of it.

My doctor told me a story that I now see was not wrong but rather simplified. He said, "we know why people feel this way. Sometimes something goes wrong in people's brains. There is a natural chemical imbalance. All we need to do is give you a drug to get your chemicals back to normal. So he gave me an antidepressant.

And I felt a lot better for a while, I had a real boost, but then the depression came back. So they gave me higher and higher doses until, for 13 years, I was taking the maximum dose possible but still had a lot of pain. So, I started to wonder: "I'm doing everything they tell me to do; Why do I keep feeling like this? "

I interviewed leading scientific experts and people who have been through depression everywhere. I learned that there is scientific evidence for nine factors that lead to our depression. Two of them are, in fact, in our biology.

Your genes can make you more sensitive to these problems, and there are real changes in the brain that occur when you get depressed that can make it harder to get out. But most of the factors that have been shown to cause depression and anxiety are not in our biology.

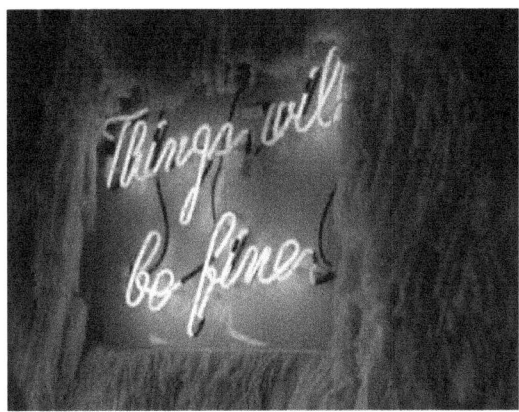

For example, if you are lonely, you are much more likely to become depressed. If you are in control at work, you are much more likely to get depressed. If you don't interact with the natural world, you are much more likely to become depressed. These are factors of the way we live, and once you understand them, a very different set of solutions opens up that must be offered alongside the option of drugs.

We all know that we have natural physical needs. You need food, shelter, water, and clean air. There is equally strong evidence that all human beings have natural psychological needs. You need to feel that you belong. You need to feel that your life has meaning and purpose.

This culture we have built is good at many things, but we are becoming less and less good at meeting people's deep underlying psychological needs.

Some part of my book asks what the unmet psychological needs leading to this epidemic of depression and anxiety are. And so how can we begin to build a culture that meets those needs?

Our clinical system is created to respond mainly to biological problems. There are some real biological causes of depression, but they exist alongside and interact with these huge psychological and social causes.

I'll start by giving you an example. Everyone knows that junk food has taken over our diet and made us physically sick. I'm not saying this with any superiority. I came here from McDonald's. But there is equally strong evidence that some kind of junk values have taken over our minds and made us mentally ill.

For thousands of years, philosophers have said, "If you think life is about money, and status, and display, you're going to feel like shit." It is not an exact quote from Confucius, but it is the gist of what he said. But strangely, no one had scientifically proven this until an amazing man I met named Professor Tim.

His research suggests crucial insights. The more you think that life is about buying things and showing them and how you see yourself to other people, the more likely you are to get depressed and anxious in a significant amount. And as a society, we have become *much* more driven by these forces.

At first, this seems pretty obvious. Everyone knows that you will not lie on your deathbed and think about all the likes you have on Instagram and all the shoes you bought. You will think of moments of love and connection.

But, as Professor Tim told me, we live in a machine designed so that we neglect what is important in life. We are constantly bombarded with messages telling us to look for happiness in the wrong places.

Professor Tim wanted to find out if we can disrupt that machine. He did an experiment in which he had people come together, once every few weeks, for months, to talk about the times when they have found meaning and purpose in their lives.

For some people, it was playing music or running on the beach with their children. The group was designed to ask – how can you spend more of your life on these things and less on these junk values?

They showed that only this experience led to a significant change in people's values. It alienated them from the forces that caused so much depression.

These are causes that go far beyond our biology, and our current medical system is not good at responding to non-biological causes.

I think it is too simplistic to say that these causes "respond to the dynamics of capitalist life."

First of all, several of them, like childhood traumas, have nothing to do with capitalism. And secondly, in communist societies like the Soviet Union and North Korea, there was an enormous amount of depression, despair, and anxiety, almost certainly more than in our societies.

Any kind of economy – capitalist, communist, social-democratic – can fail to meet people's underlying human needs if it doesn't work well. The core problem is that many of the deepest needs of people as humans are not being met by how our society works right now.

But to address your question. If you don't understand what causes a problem, it is really difficult to solve. So far, most people have been offered a very simplistic story about their depression. They say it is solely and entirely a problem with your brain chemistry.

That only leads to one solution: drugs. The drugs give some relief, but for most, sadly, they are not solving the problem in the long run. The best scientific research shows that most people who take chemical antidepressants become depressed again. So, we need to have a deeper understanding of the problem to expand the menu of solutions.

For example?

In 2000, a South African psychiatrist named Derek Summerfield was in Cambodia doing some research on the psychological effects of unexploded landmines, at a time when chemical antidepressants were being marketed for the first time in the country.

Local doctors didn't know much about these drugs, so they asked Summerfield to explain them. When he finished, they explained that they didn't need these new chemicals because they already had antidepressants.

Puzzled, Derek asked them to explain, hoping they would tell him about some local herbal remedy. Instead, they told him about something quite different.

They told him a story about a farmer they had treated. He was working in the rice fields, and one day he stepped on a landmine and had his leg blown off. They put an artificial limb on him, and eventually, he went back to work.

But it is very painful to work when your joint is underwater, and returning to the field where it was blown up made him very anxious. He became deeply depressed.

Doctors and his neighbors sat down with this man and talked about his life and his problems. They realized that even with his new artificial limb, his old job was too difficult, that he was constantly stressed and in physical pain, and that these things combined to simply want to stop living.

His interlocutors had an idea. They suggested that he work as a milkman, a job that would cause less pain for his false leg and produce fewer disturbing memories. They believed that he was perfectly capable of making the switch. So they bought him a cow.

In the months and years that followed, his life changed. His depression, which was once deep, lifted. Cambodian doctors told Dr. Summerfield, "You see, doctor, the cow was an antidepressant."

Over time, I came to believe that this little scene in Southeast Asia, which at first sounds a bit quirky, actually represents, in a distilled way, a change in perspective that many of us have to make if we want to progress.

Only because they understood the cause of the farmer's depression could they find the solution. So we have to ask ourselves: what is causing our depression, and what is the cow for that?

I have seen the answer to this question put into practice. We are the loneliest society in the history of mankind. A recent study asked Americans, "how many people know you well?" Half of them said no one.

It's not that bad in America, but it's getting worse. I spent a lot of time talking to a man named Professor John in Chicago, the world's leading expert on solitude. He said to me – why do we exist? Everyone in this room, all of us?

One reason is that our ancestors in the savannas of Africa were very good at one thing. They weren't bigger than the animals they shot down; they weren't faster than the animals they shot down, but they were much better at grouping together and cooperating. Just as bees evolved to live in a hive, humans evolved to live in a tribe.

We are the first humans to try to dissolve our tribes.

But there is a solution. One of my heroes is a doctor named Sam Everington. He is a general practitioner in a poor area of East London, where I lived for a long time, and he was very uncomfortable. He had many patients who came to him with depression, and like me, he is not opposed to chemical antidepressants, which for some people, are an advantage, but he could see that for many of his patients, they were not solving their problems. So one day, he decided to try something different.

A woman came into his office named Lisa Cunningham. I met her later. Lisa had been locked up at home with paralyzing depression and anxiety for seven years. He had barely left his house. Sam said, "Don't worry, I'll keep giving you these drugs." But I'm also going to prescribe something else.

There was an area behind the medical office suite that was just a bare lot. Sam said to Lisa, "What I would like you to do is come and go, a few times a week, to this lot, and meet with a group of other depressed and anxious people to find something meaningful to do together."

The first time the group met, Lisa was physically ill. But the group started talking, and they asked: what can we do? And they decided that they were going to build a garden. They were people from central East London like me who didn't know anything about gardening. So they started reading books, watching videos.

They began to put their fingers in the ground. They began to learn the rhythms of the seasons. There is much evidence that exposure to the natural world is a very powerful antidepressant.

But they started to do something even more important. They began to form a tribe. They began to form a group. They began to worry about each other. If one of them didn't show up, they'd go looking for them.

As Lisa told me, when the garden began to bloom, we began to bloom. This approach is called social prescribing, and there is a growing body of evidence showing that it produces substantial drops in depression and anxiety.

In this culture, we are constantly told, when we feel anxious or depressed, to be you. Be yourself. As if individualism is what we should be looking for. But, what depression taught me is, don't be you. Don't be yourself. Let's be us. Let's be us. What we should aspire to is to be part of a tribe.

The most important thing is to explain to people that if you are depressed or anxious, that you are not weak. He is not mad. He is not, in general, a machine with broken parts. He is a human being with unmet needs and what he deserves is love and support to meet those deepest needs. Once you understand this, you can begin to solve some of the problems that cause so much depression.

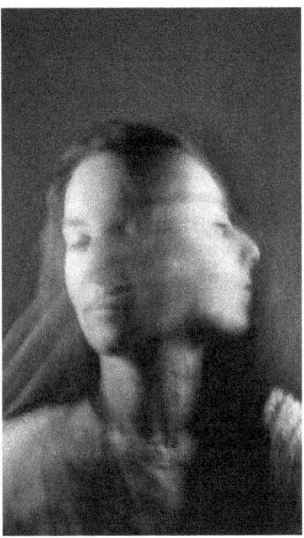

We can ask people if they hate their job. There is strong evidence that human beings need to feel that our lives have meaning, that we are doing something with a purpose that makes a difference. It is a natural psychological need. But between 2011 and 2012, the Gallup polling company conducted the most detailed study ever conducted of how people feel that we spend most of our waking lives doing our paid work.

They found that 13% of people say they are "committed" to their work, find it meaningful, and look forward to it. 63% say they are "not engaged," which is defined as "sleepwalking on their workday." And 24% are "actively offline" – they hate it.

Most of the depressed and anxious people I know, I realized, are in the 87% who don't like their job. So, I started inquiring to see if there is any evidence that this could be related to depression. It turned out that an Australian scientist named Michael Marmott had made a breakthrough in answering this question in the 1970s.

He wanted to investigate what causes stress in the workplace, and he believed he had found the perfect laboratory to discover the answer: British civil service, based in Whitehall.

This small army of bureaucrats and officials was divided into nineteen different layers, from the Permanent Secretary at the top to the typists at the bottom. What I wanted to know, at first, was:

Everyone told him: you're wasting your time. The boss is going to be more stressed because he has more responsibility. But when Michael published his results, he revealed that the exact opposite was true. The lower an employee is in the hierarchy, the higher their stress level, and the likelihood of having a heart attack. Now I wanted to know: why?

And that's when, after two more years studying officials, he discovered the biggest factor. It turns out that if you have no control over your work, you are much more likely to get stressed and, more importantly, to get depressed.

Humans have an innate need to feel that what we are doing daily is meaningful. When you are in control, you cannot create meaning from your work.

Suddenly, the depression of many of my friends, even those with fancy jobs, who spend most of their waking hours feeling controlled and unappreciated, started to seem like not a problem with their brains, but a problem with their environments.

I learned that there are many causes of depression like this. But my journey was not simply about finding the reasons why we feel so bad. The core was figuring out how we can feel better and find real, long-lasting antidepressants that work for most of us, beyond the pill packs we've been offered so often as the only menu item for the depressed and the anxious. We have to deal with the deeper issues that are causing all this anguish.

You decided that you consciously and deliberately wanted to take steps to be a happier person. Let's say you decided to spend two hours a day being happier. They wanted to find out. Does doing that make you happier? Works? They studied this in four countries: the United States, Russia, Japan, and Taiwan.

And what they found out was that at first, it looked really weird. If you consciously try to make yourself happier in the United States, you don't become happier. But in other countries, if you try to make yourself happier, you do it. They were averages. There were exceptions.

Why would that be? What is happening here? They went and studied it more. They found that in America, in general, if you try to make yourself happier, you do something for yourself. You buy something; you work harder for a promotion, you treat yourself, whatever it is.

In other countries, in general, if you try to make yourself happier, you do something for another person, your friends, your family, your community. So, we have an implicitly individualistic story about happiness. They have an implicit collectivist story about happiness. And it turns out that our vision of happiness doesn't work. Some kind of individualists would have died in the savannas of Africa.

And after he explained it to me, I realized that my story about happiness had been wrong for a long time. When I felt these painful feelings approaching, I met them with some individual accomplishment, buying something for myself, doing something "awesome" at work, doing some kind of external accomplishment. And it rarely worked. It rarely made me happier.

When I feel those painful feelings coming (and sometimes I do), I try to do something for someone else. It can be as simple as leaving my phone at home, visiting them, and listening to them. In a society where people are so lonely, being heard is an incredible gift.

And this simple change, of realizing that my happiness can only come from boosting others' happiness, has had a strong effect on me.

All of that is very important. To progress, we need to start by changing our understanding of what depression and anxiety are. There are very real biological contributions to depression and anxiety.

But if we allow biology to become the big picture, implicitly telling people: your pain means nothing. It's a wiring problem in your brain, like a glitch in a computer program.

I could only begin to change my life when I learned that your depression is not a problem. It is a sign. Your pain makes sense. You feel that way for reasons, and those reasons can be addressed. It took me a long time to conclude, but the message from the scientists and the crisis around us is increasingly clear. We have to stop insulting these signals and start listening to them because they tell us something we need to hear.

As a culture, we have become deeply individualistic. It has trained us to seek happiness in all the wrong places.

I had a pretty bad depression for a long time, from my teens. I experienced pretty severe abuse from an adult as a child. I never wanted to think about this or talk about it. I didn't want to give this individual power over me now.

In writing my book, I interviewed leading experts who have shown how childhood traumas can cause depression and all kinds of problems in adults, like obesity and addiction.

And they taught me something very important that they had found in their research. It is not the abuse that destroys you. It is a shame of abuse. And if you can find safe places to release the shame you feel, that can free you from your depression.

People who suffer abuse in childhood tend to internalize the voice of their abuser. They think that they do not deserve to be treated with love and care. A safe and loving connection that helps you release your shame helps release those abusive voices from your mind.

Evidence shows that reducing shame heals you deeply and can reduce your depression and anxiety.

For more than 30 years, we have told, as a culture, a primal story about depression and anxiety, and that story has come to dominate the discussion.

When I was a teenager, I went to my doctor and explained that I felt the anguish coming out of me uncontrollably, like a foul smell. He told me a story. He said that depression is caused by the spontaneous lack of a chemical in the brain called serotonin. I simply needed to take some medications to raise my serotonin levels to a normal level.

Recently, a young friend of one of my nephews, not much older than I was when I was first diagnosed, went to his doctor and asked for help with his depression. Your doctor told you that you had a problem with *dopamine* in your brain. In 20 years, all that has changed is the name of the chemical.

I believed and predicted this story for more than a decade. But when I started researching the causes of depression and anxiety for my book, I was surprised to find leading scientific organizations saying that this approach was based on a misunderstanding of science. There are actual biological factors that contribute to depression, but they are far from the whole story.

I learned that the World Health Organization explained in 2011: "Mental health occurs socially: the presence or absence of mental health is above all a social indicator and therefore requires social as well as individual solutions."

The United Nations, in its official statement on the occasion of World Health Day in 2017, said that "the dominant biomedical narrative on depression" is based on "the biased and selective use of research results" that "cause more harm than good, undermine the right to health and must be abandoned. There is a "growing evidence base," said the UN authors, that there are deeper causes of depression, so while there is some role for drugs, we need to stop using them "to address issues that are closely related to social problems. We need to move from "focusing on" chemical imbalances "to focusing on" power imbalances."

At first, I was puzzled by statements like this, which went against everything I had been told. So I spent three years interviewing the world's leading scientists on these issues to understand what is going on in places where despair in our culture is worst, from Cleveland to Sao Paulo, and where the incidence of despair is minor, including Amish communities.

I learned that there is broad agreement among scientists that there are three types of causes of depression and anxiety and that all three occur, to varying degrees, in all depressed and anxious people. The causes are: biological (like your genes), psychological (how you think of yourself), and social (the broader ways we live together).

Very few people dispute this. But when it comes to communicating with the public and offering help, psychological solutions have been increasingly neglected, and environmental solutions have been almost totally ignored.

When we understand this problem differently, we can start to find real solutions.

"And here you are living, despite it all." – Rupi Kaur.

This book aims to make known the reality of mental health and basic guidelines that you have to take into account in the performance of all those tasks, which as an individual, are entrusted to you in this area.

Keep in mind that the key to success lies in the bond, the ability to share emotional time and space, accompany what goes beyond the task, where the center is the person attended, and its context.

Do not forget that you are not alone on this path, which is quite a team of which you are part, the one that is focused on following the objective: to keep our mental health in check and improve the quality of life of people affected by it.

We are all in this together.

Chapter 1: "I'm like you even if you don't know it."

Mental health is essentially defined as a state of emotional, mental, and social well-being. It affects the way we think, feel, and act. It determines our interaction with life. How we handle difficult situations, how we interact with other people, and make decisions.

But, the concept of mental health is not absolute. Not having a recognized mental disorder does not necessarily indicate that we will always fail at mental health.

The concept of health is not in black and white – you have it, or you don't have it. It is a matter of degrees. In life, we pass, and we will go through different moments, where we will find different states of physical health and mental health.

We must pay attention and care to our health in a comprehensive way. The type of difficulties and how we face them will determine the appearance or not of some emotional or psychological disorder, and this may be of different types and intensities.

For all this, the concept of mental health should be a natural concept, like physical health, without prejudice or stigma. We all will go through times when we will experience a problem, but that does not mean that we are the problem.

I like the slogan of the Spanish Mental Health Confederation recent campaign on World Mental Health Day: "I'm like you even if you don't know it." It comes to remind us that when we talk about having or not having mental health, we are all in the same "boat." The figures offered by the different epidemiological studies tell us about what mental health is like in the world are staggering.

A European study that was carried out in 2010 that included 30 countries showed data that 38.2%, that is, 164 million people in Europe, had some mental disorder at the time of the study.

It is also essential to pay attention to the data on mental disorders in children and adolescents. Some epidemiological studies indicate that between 7 and 25% of minors meet the criteria for a psychiatric diagnosis.

The most common mental problems or disorders are anxiety, insomnia, and depression. The five mental disorders with the greatest impact are dysthymia, major depressive episode, post-traumatic stress disorders, panic disorder, and social phobia.

Although certain efforts are made, and in the Declaration of Helsinki (European Declaration, 2006), it is urged to promote a shift from attention to mental health services, we still have much to do.

For now, only a small fraction of people with mental health problems receive treatment, and in many cases, with delay or ineffective treatments.

Another large part of the population does not even know that they have a mental illness. As institutions work to improve these care levels, what can we do for ourselves, our friends, and family?

What can we do for our mental health?

First, we can learn to detect our problems and be more aware of them. Having information and more self-awareness is the first step in solving our difficulties.

Many people manage to feel that they are "bad" even "awful." Still, they do not identify this high discomfort with suffering from some disorder, such as depression, a personality disorder, an eating disorder, or an obsessive disorder.

It may seem surprising to us, but it is the reality, and I see it frequently in the office and my environment. Too many people attend to their difficulties with an "I'll get over it" or an "I'm like this."

Either they never attend to those problems, or they delay their attention for up to five or more years. And in the course of the problem, they strive and fight to be better. From the knowledge they have at their fingertips, they apply intuition or allow themselves to be advised by friends, and they live day by day, facing symptoms that make their life.

On many occasions, a true ordeal.

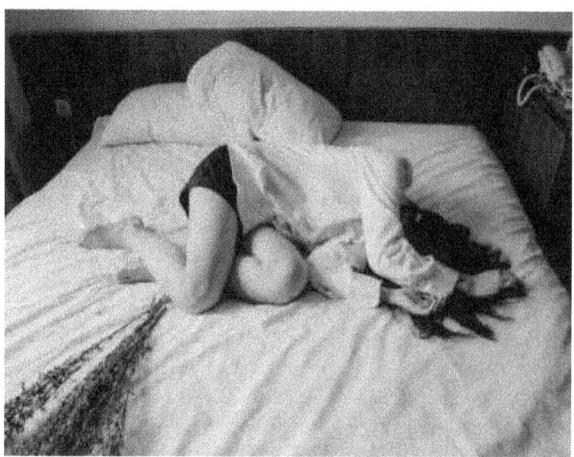

Thus, the first important question in mental health is to have adequate and sufficient information to acquire knowledge and be aware, identify, and prevent problems.

If they are aware of their illness, their problems and have decided to go to a psychologist, psychologist, or psychiatrist. Many people have decided to go to a psychologist, psychologist, or psychiatrist to deal with them.

Even though they have not chosen to be ill and have not made any conscious decisions that have caused their illness, they feel guilty and ashamed and suffer isolation and the effects of a stigma that remains today associated with mental illness.

People naturally accept having a physical illness. We do not feel guilty about it. We share it, we express it, they understand us, and with it, we obtain support from others, and we feel relieved and accompanied.

We all hear people talking about their illnesses as part of the natural, daily conversations in their life. However, in general, we are ashamed; we feel weak, inferior, guilty, incapable, and we hide it.

Throughout these years, more than half of the people I know and talk to, at some point have expressed to me with great sadness, also with helplessness and above all with feelings of loneliness, that they could not share their psychological problems, that they did not understand them, and that they carried their illness in silence, for fear of being seen as weak, of rejection, of dismissal, and also for fear of the banal responses of others, devoid of empathy, generated from the lack of "culture and knowledge about mental health."

Phrases like: "What you have to do is go out and have fun." "It's that you don't make an effort." "You lack the will." "Happiness is a choice." The worst thing is that these comments often convince those who suffer from mental disorders that this is the case.

Having a mental health problem cannot be a secret or embarrassment, but a challenge to achieve our balance.

We all have a person by our side with a mental health problem, or we will have one, according to the figures provided by epidemiological studies. We may have one or more mental health problems throughout our lives. It is time to prepare and move forward in the knowledge of mental illness and understand those who suffer from it.

Let us ask with respect and without judging, seek information from good sources, listen without giving solutions that we do not have, give only support, that in these difficult moments do not feel alone or alone.

A mental health problem cannot be a secret, nor an embarrassment, but a challenge.

It would be good if, from these reflections, we move forward with a mind clear of fear and prejudice towards the construction of better mental health, ours, and everyone's. We develop our emotional capacities to enjoy ourselves and others, our partners and family, and achieve the harmony and well-being we all deserve.

When we enter a hospital or a health center and see the mental health area signposted, or even when we go down the street and see a psychology center advertised, what is the first thing that comes to mind? What do we associate mental health with?

If any of the meanings of the expression "being crazy" is included in your answer, I think we are on the same page.

"Madness" an image full of prejudices

I have been talking to psychologists for years. I have always believed that progress and knowledge would remove prejudices, stereotypes, and stigmas from the field of mental health. And although there has been a significant advance, I still find people who resist going to a psychologist's consultation. If they do, they maintain modest secrecy with their family and friends. Everything is to avoid being considered "crazy"!

The professionals who work in mental health have special care using the word "madness." It is not that we have any taboo on the term, but that they are aware of the "imagery" that around this expression they have created Literature, cinema, or even history itself, with those "controversial" biographies of some "illustrious characters."

In short, everything has contributed to the fact that when we detect any sign that something in our way of thinking or our emotions is not "normal" – and later, we will speak of "normality" – we feel enormous discomfort and fear.

Curiously, in these times, there is a concern that quite the contrary, we usually boast about: physical health. We tell all our family and friends that we go to the gym, that we have started a super diet, that we train our body, and even – if our pockets allow it – that we have a "personal trainer."

And nobody judges us for it. They are more likely to congratulate us.

Doesn't it seem paradoxical to you that we don't feel any shame in training our body, and instead, it doesn't seem convenient to train our mind? Don't you think that we should speak with the same naturalness of aspiring to good mental health to good physical health?

And I can't resist asking one more question. Don't you think that if we have a specialist in the human body for this physical health training, we shouldn't have a specialist of the mind, a psychologist, to train mental health, which is at least the same or more complex?

Aspiring to improve our resources, capacities, and emotional abilities mean learning to think better and relate better. In short, to live happier and more satisfied is not a "crazy" aspiration.

Who goes to see a psychologist?

People come to consultations to train their ability to speak in public, improve their "sleep hygiene," relate and communicate socially in a natural way, be assertive and honest with themselves, have a fuller sexual life, or improve their ability to lead human teams in positions of responsibility.

Do you think these people, with these aspirations, are crazy? Of course not.

There are many examples of people who have adequate functioning in their day to day but decide to request help to improve, change, reflect, decide, etc. In short, take action and overcome new goals. Because every day we are clearer about our well-being, our happiness depends primarily on us, on our behavior, attitude, and thinking.

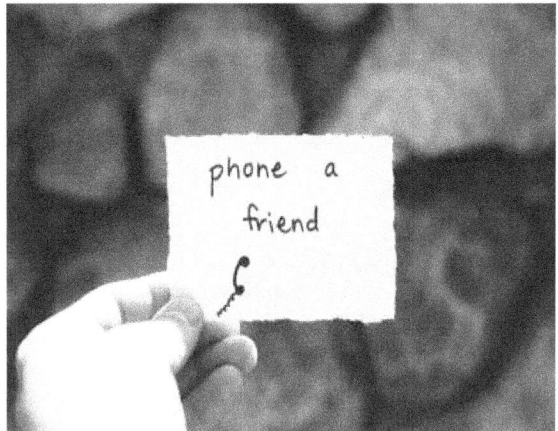

And here a new prejudice appears: "It's that I'm like that, I can't change."

On many occasions, we believe that happiness depends on our environment, the situation we live in, whether we have health, a partner, money, or work. But did you know that this variable – the situation – only influences our happiness by 10%? And the remaining 90%?

Let's see some data on the perception of happiness.

50% depends on our genetics, our natural tendencies, personality variables, and our biology. And 40% depends on us, on our behavior, on our coping, on our way of handling emotions.

And I'm going to tell you a little secret, in that 40% is where happiness is perceived more intensely. In other words, when we manage to be happy thanks to something that we have achieved, and not something that is given to us, the feeling of happiness is much fuller.

Each of us can increase our well-being, our happiness, by 40%. Don't you think it's worth it? Don't you think all the help is good in this challenge?

What is psychology for?

Part of psychology professionals' work is to guide, discover resources, train, and direct for your great personal challenge, just like when you prepare a long-distance race and have a coach.

Psychologists treat psychopathology, anxiety disorders, depression, personality disorders, or eating behavior disorders. Still, the reasons for consultation not associated with disorders but with imbalances and daily problems of our day are persistent: insomnia, relationship problems, smoking cessation, grief, decision-making, poor control of anger, communication problems with children, self-esteem.

In short, Clinical Psychology is not only science at the service of pathologies. It also has the purpose of helping you discover your personality components and guide you so that you decide what to do with them, what to improve, complement, and overcome. It helps you to become the owner of your emotions, but not by blocking or avoiding them – that's impossible, they have a fundamental role in our life – the goal is to increase the perception of control over them and decide how to act, being fully aware of what we feel. We do, taking control of our life, without being like a weather vane carried away by the wind, by any wind.

There are many myths related to the profession. A few myths about psychology and psychologists:

1. Only those who are weak need help.
2. Psychologists can guess your thoughts. They are like fortune tellers.
3. All those who go to the psychologist are crazy.
4. All psychology professionals have a bad head. They are weird.
5. They brainwash you.
6. They tell you what to do.
7. All psychological treatments are long.
8. If you stop going to the psychologist, your problems come back.

Psychologists are health professionals who are experts in behavior and emotions. They provide strategies to acquire emotional skills and resources that improve the physical and psychological health of the people, always respecting patients' decisions, motivations, and needs. But, what is the line that separates normal from abnormal? When do I know I need help? When do emotions become a problem? When emotions are a sign that something is wrong:

- If they generate psychological discomfort several times a day for an extended period.
- If emotions generate a high physiological activation and it is maintained over time.
- If they negatively affect our health.
- If it hinders our performance.
- If they generate maladaptive behavior (increased arguments, isolation, absenteeism from work, substance abuse, bingeing, etc.).
- If we perceive not having control over them, they dominate us and condition our day to day.

Do not forget that for everyone, knowing our limits is a significant discovery in life. Demanding the right help at the right time is not a sign of weakness, but of intelligence, and also of strength and courage.

Cognitive behavioral therapy. The choice of treatment

"I'm going to improve; I want to go to a psychologist, but... where?" What will they do? How will they do it?

I know, I know that deciding to improve is a great advance. I know that deciding to go to a psychologist is a first step that shows conviction and motivation.

But I also know that from that moment on, questions arise that are not always, and not for all or all, easy to answer: Which psychology center do I go to? What do I have to ask? What type of professional in psychology should I choose? What is this Cognitive Behavioral Therapy thing I've heard about?

The first visit to a psychologist or psychologist is not easy. Many and very diverse are the reasons, feelings, and weaknesses present in those who consider taking the step of receiving psychological treatment.

A feeling that is practically in all of the people who live this experience is that of insecurity. Insecurity in the face of the emotional discomfort they suffer, the impossibility of handling it on their own, and the doubt of what they will find when receiving therapy. As will be? What will they tell me? Will it help me?

In the moments in which we perceive ourselves with more fragility, looking for stable, specific, reliable support is usually the first step, necessary to regain the feeling of control in our day to day, the feeling of security. And there a fundamental question arises:

Can we entrust this professional support to any type of psychological therapy and any psychologist or psychologist? The answer, without a doubt, is the intuited one: no.

I have written this section with a clear objective: to answer the most frequently asked questions – five specifically – asked by people who attend first sessions or take the preliminary interview.

What is cognitive behavioral, psychological treatment?

Cognitive behavioral therapy is a type of psychological therapy that is not based on intuition or personal interpretation of the psychologist or psychologist who directs, but a methodology, a defined system, whose effectiveness and guarantees clinics have been demonstrated and supported by scientific studies.

In this clinical system, the first phase is essential: an evaluation.

The psychological evaluation is carried out through various procedures, the scope, and variety, which will be determined by the reasons for consultation or the aspects that the psychologist appreciates in the first sessions.

Some of these procedures are clinical interviews, evaluation tests or questionnaires, and self-records that the person performs.

Now in which the two active subjects in the treatment:

- A person seeking change.
- A Psychologist who directs it, they agree that it has been clearly understood what is happening, why it is happening, and why the problem remains, it is time to continue with the next phase of treatment: how to change it.

In most psychological practices, they dedicate a session to deliver and explain a written report. All the conclusions drawn in the evaluation phase are exposed.

Such a report includes an explanatory model that details the relationship between the main processes involved in the problem, a series of specific and valuable objectives, and a treatment plan to achieve these objectives.

1. **What is the choice of some treatment techniques based on and not others?**

And again, I must insist that treatment techniques are never chosen based on the professional's intuition or personal preference. In cognitive behavioral therapy, those techniques and clinical tools are chosen, which have proven to be more effective in changing the dysfunctional processes identified in the evaluation phase.

Comparing it with other health processes, if you have fallen and your arm hurts, I would not do a blood test to evaluate a possible fracture: I would perform an x-ray because it is the appropriate and ideal evaluation procedure for the problem.

And if we see a fracture, I would not prescribe exercises because "I know that will help you" I would recommend immobilization of the arm because studies show that an initial period of immobilization is necessary after a fracture of these characteristics.

In cognitive behavioral therapy, saving distances, we work along the same lines. There is a form of evaluation and treatments established as the most suitable and most effective for each process or psychological problem.

Those of us who work in the Health area have no doubts: let us work with the most adequate and efficient scientific procedures, and not with others!

As Llobell, Frías Navarro, and Monterde i Bor (2004) say: The wide proliferation of psychological treatments that currently exist requires control of their quality and effects.

Not everything goes well when applying a psychological technique or procedure to a person with a series of problems.

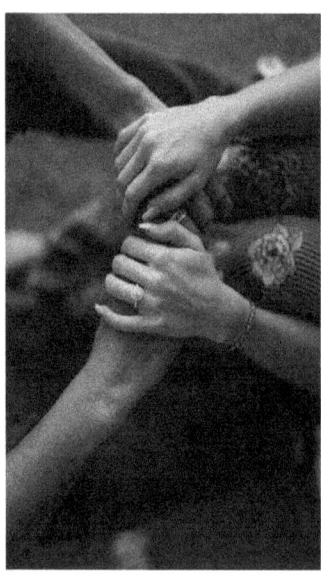

2. **What is the normal frequency of cognitive behavioral therapy? Will I go every week? When and how does it end?**

The frequency of sessions in cognitive behavioral therapy is not something improvised either. Studies have shown that in the first phase, a weekly frequency is the one that obtains the best results and does so in the shortest time.

When the change process begins to stabilize (the proposed objectives begin to be partially achieved), the sessions are separated (once every two weeks, for example). And when the goals are practically achieved, the sessions are even further apart (once a month at first, then once every 2-3 months). In the last phase, called follow-up, what is sought is:

- Strengthen the learned processes that have led to the change.
- Prevent possible relapses.

After some follow-up sessions, the process is finished.

3. **What if psychological treatment is not helping me?**

Since a treatment plan with objectives is established, from time to time, it is advisable for the psychologist and the patient to spend time sharing and contrasting how and to what extent the objectives are being met.

This sharing is very useful to consolidate and reinforce and reorient, redirect, or introduce the necessary treatment changes.

The fundamental thing is that the person knows that the objective is to overcome the problem and make his change. For this, you will have the professional attention of the psychologist or psychologist who directs your treatment and all the clinical resources, information, and support.

4. **How long does a cognitive behavioral treatment last?**

It depends. Different manifestations are clear warnings that it is convenient to seek professional help: loss of control, feeling of hopelessness, blockage in the face of a situation that we cannot face, continuous negative thoughts.

The duration of the treatment will be determined. On one hand, what is the reason or the problem for which the person goes to psychological treatment: anxiety? Phobias? Emotional dissatisfaction without locating an exact cause? Difficulties in decision-making?

How long have you been living with this problem, and how it has evolved and taken root in aspects not only personal but also family, professional, etc.

We must understand that psychological treatment aims to produce changes and that making any change is a process that requires actions that transform aspects of our life, which sometimes costs a lot to modify.

Another aspect that influences the duration of treatment is the dynamics of clinical work itself. How much motivation is there in the process? How much involvement in the exercises proposed between sessions?

How much adjustment on the part of the professional to the techniques and treatments proven to be effective? Cognitive behavioral treatment is not a long-term therapy. On the contrary, it is considered an effective and brief treatment.

The important thing is that the treatment duration does not violate or detract from the planned objectives. The person always has clear and precise information on how and why psychological therapy is being developed at that rate.

So far, I have tried to answer what I consider the five most frequent questions about cognitive behavioral therapy, but there are others that I do not want to miss.

What if I am not sure about the orientation? What else will benefit me? How can I compare it with other options? What can I do to decide where to go?

The process of choosing a psychology center and professional is something especially difficult. It is common to reference someone close, which is usually an essential criterion in our choice, but is it enough?

Some steps before making this decision will be very useful for you:

1. **Get informed**. Decide what type of therapy you want to receive. Be interested in the type of treatments practiced in the centers where you consult, and ask for information about how the clinical procedure is in that therapy and if it is the best scientifically supported for your situation or personal problem. Question: What and how is it done? Is it the most effective? Why?

2. **Get up close**. When in doubt, have a first contact with the center and the professional you would work with. Before you take the step of starting treatment, go for an initial interview. In that contact, you can receive precious information about how the treatment will be and how you have felt talking to that person in whom you would place your trust.

3. **It requires the necessary health accreditations**. Choose a center with guarantees, where all psychologists have accreditation from the Official College of Psychologists; the center has all the pertinent permits for health activity; that at the administration level, it responds to all legal requirements: billing, data protection law, etc. All these guarantees are not only an expression of seriousness and rigor. They usually show well-organized and defined work systems, with protocols and control procedures that guarantee you a quality service.

4. **Look for confidence**. Choose with conviction where and with whom you want to work. Even before deciding, from the first contact, express your doubts, fears, and uncertainties about the process. See if the environment, the professional, and the type of treatment they offer you give you the conviction that you will need in the process.

5. **Seek safety**. It is legitimate to demand good treatment. But beyond this, make it easy! Choose professionals who have those qualities that you consider necessary. It's your choice! Intelligence, responsibility, good manners, commitment, tenacity, dedication, sensitivity, empathy, closeness, respect.

Emotional mind: adaptation and satisfaction

I'm going to ask you to think about situations that have made you feel bad. But first I want to ask you: do you consider yourself a person with good emotional skills?

Surely, in the last few weeks, you have been through some unpleasant experiences. Someone has not gone to an important appointment. You have not felt capable in the face of difficulty. Your child has reacted inappropriately with you.

You feel that your partner is less involved in your relationship, someone has told you something that you have felt unfair, they have rejected in a job interview, you feel displaced by some friends, you can't control something important that you want to change, someone tested positive for COVID-19...

What did you feel, with what intensity, how long did the discomfort caused by the situation persist? Did it scare you to feel bad? What did you do to stop feeling disgusted? What did you do to resolve the situation?

Take a moment before you start reading this section, write down the current situations that have affected you, and identify the following elements:

1. Situation (what happened).
2. Emotion (how you felt).
3. Thoughts (what ideas came up). Interpretation of the facts and the emotions that are felt.
4. Conduct (what did you do).

With this simple technique, you will observe your emotional states and identify your limitations or strengths when facing what happens to you in your day to day.

It will allow you to reflect on what aspects influence your emotional experiences, obtain information that you may have overlooked, and promote learning and adaptation.

The value of emotional competencies

Emotions play a fundamental role in the processes of adaptation to changes – desired or unforeseen. Also, in our activities' daily performance, in the learning processes, interpersonal interactions, and of course, in our well-being and health.

The confinement and health crisis has been a challenge for most people regarding the management of their emotions. We have implemented strategies of all kinds, physical and psychological, to promote a better adaptation and face uncertainty, reduce chronic interpersonal sources of gratification, promote pleasant emotions, despite difficulties, and devise ways to reduce or manage stress.

All of this has tested our emotional stamina. But it has also allowed us to become aware of our ability to mobilize resources aimed at managing complex emotions, organizing our priorities and needs, and trying to solve obstacles in these circumstances.

We have learned many things, we have had the opportunity to observe and know our strengths and abilities. The moments of introspection have most likely revealed aspects of our emotional management and coping that could be improved.

Life constantly puts us before a dilemma: lock ourselves and deepen in suffering, or adopt a resilient and learning approach, adapting to the situation in a productive way for our emotional well-being.

If we decide on the second option, we will need our emotional skills.

Emotional competencies can be defined as a set of knowledge, abilities, skills, and attitudes necessary to understand, express, and regulate emotional phenomena appropriately (p.22, Bisquerra, 2003).

Emotional competencies have become increasingly important as protective factors for personal and social health and well-being. They are considered predictors of success in academic life and at all levels of adult life (Ibarrola, 2014).

In the last two decades, they are increasingly valued and required in work and professional environments due to the constant technological transformations, which entail an effort to adapt, learn, and manage information.

Also, at the interpersonal level, emotional competencies are decisive. Society is increasingly complex and changing: multiculturalism, geographical mobility, globalization, multinationalism of personal relationships.

Emotional education in educational contexts is gaining relevance given the growing recognition of the role of emotions in teaching and learning processes and the positive impact on the development of people's potentialities and their psychological, physical, and social well-being.

What are emotional competencies? What are the main ones? Why are they so valuable? How are they learned and trained?

Emotions and affective states greatly influence many cognitive processes such as reasoning, attention, memory, and perception, fundamental in the processing of information.

Emotions can facilitate, distort, or inhibit central processes in the acquisition, assimilation, storage, and retrieval of information (De Aparicio, 2009).

Imagine that when you get home after a difficult day, where you are upset, angry, you see that the instructions you gave before leaving for work have not been followed.

Another day you would care less, but today: you see everything worse than it is (attention), you misinterpret what they tell you (information processing), and you remember – even if you don't want to – the time's something similar has happened to you (your memory is consistent with your state of mind).

But what would happen if you came happy, after a good day, and found yourself facing the same situation?

Emotions are psychophysiological reactions – cognitive, physiological, and behavioral responses – in response to external or internal situations, events, and demands, which predispose to action, through a rapid organization to face the experience.

For example, when we feel jealous – of a partner, co-workers, or friends – our body tenses, our pulse quickens, we activate our attention, and analyze events related to the situation. We act, we seek information, we value, we interpret. Not all people react in the same way to the same situation. Then there are different ways of dealing with the same situation and different emotional consequences.

Knowing how we react, what we feel, how we can regulate the different, more automatic emotional responses to improve our thinking and disposition to certain tasks or situations relevant to our well-being are emotional competencies that support emotional intelligence.

Thus, the result of doing things in an emotionally intelligent way would be, accepting jealousy as an emotion we can have, observing and understanding why it is, and acting to minimize jealousy, being realistic, and not damaging a good relationship due to unfounded assumptions.

Emotional competencies: the basis of emotional intelligence

The concept of emotional intelligence became popular with Daniel Goleman's "bestseller" (1995). However, it was Salovey and Mayer in 1990, who coined the term emotional intelligence and proposed a model based on different emotional abilities - which is one of the most consolidated today.

Emotional intelligence for these authors consists of managing our own emotions and those of others, discriminating between them, and using the information they provide us to guide our thinking and actions (Molero, Saiz & Esteban, 1998).

In other words, emotional intelligence would be the ability to process emotional information accurately and effectively: the ability to perceive, assimilate, understand, express, and regulate emotions, own and of others (Mayer and Salovey, 1997; Mayer, Caruso and Salovey 1999; 2001).

Thus, Goleman (1998) describes it as the ability to recognize one's feelings and those of others, motivate oneself, and manage one's emotionality and emotions in interpersonal relationships.

The principles or basic emotional competencies in adequate emotional intelligence are: self-knowledge, self-control, self- motivation, empathy, social skills, assertiveness, proactivity, and creativity in the way of facing and solving problems

offers a comprehensive review of the different proposals regarding emotional competencies and proposes a model in which the different abilities are organized into five emotional competencies:

1. **Emotional awareness**

Ability to perceive, identify, and understand emotions in oneself or oneself and others through verbal and non-verbal expression.

- Facial expression.
- Voice tone.
- Body expressiveness.
- Adequate handling of emotional language.
- Empathy or understanding of the perspectives of others, get involved in their experiences.
- Read the situational and expression keys that have a degree of cultural consensus.

2. **Emotional regulation**

Ability to adequately handle emotions.

- Know the interactions between emotion, thought, and behavior.
- Expression of own emotions.
- Recognize and can regulate some feelings and emotions with a substantial impact on the behaviors they drive.
- Have skills to deal with unpleasant or uncomfortable emotions that favor the reduction in intensity, duration, and frequency of unpleasant emotions.
- In a complementary and vital way, it can self-generate and experience pleasant emotions consciously and voluntarily.

3. Emotional autonomy

This competence includes various characteristics and attitudes related to personal self-management: personal characteristics that allow external stimuli not to affect the person drastically, allowing them to be sensitive but with a certain capacity for self-protection.

- Possess positive self-esteem.
- Ability to self-motivate and get involved in various activities of life.
- Ability to take responsibility for decisions, to engage in healthy, safe, and ethical behaviors.
- Perception of emotional self-efficacy.
- Ability to resiliently face adverse situations.
- Interpersonal intelligence
- Ability to build and maintain good relationships with other people.
- Mastery of social skills, communication skills, and receptive listening.
- Ability to share emotions in a way appropriate to the relationship structure and context.
- Assertiveness.
- Prosocial and cooperative attitudes, respect, and acceptance of individual differences.
- Skills to prevent and solve problems or conflicts.
- Ability to face daily challenges and exceptional situations adaptively and responsibly, which allows us to organize life in a healthy and balanced way, contributing to experiencing satisfaction and well-being.
- The ability to set positive, achievable, and realistic goals.
- Decision-making in different areas of life.
- Seeking resources and support when necessary.
- The exercise of active, civic, responsible, critical, and committed citizenship.
- The ability to consciously enjoy well-being and try to transmit it to the people with whom you interact.

The organization in these emotional competencies will allow us to outline a framework or conceptual map for our self-knowledge, which allows us to recognize our strengths, what skills we are best at, and what our Achilles heel is.

Identifying our emotional competencies will undoubtedly be essential to begin a growth path and strengthening in the personal, professional, and social sphere.

There are five basic emotional competencies, and they are the basis of the so-called emotional intelligence. Each and every one of them is decisive for our well-being and happiness.

Sometimes we have misconceptions about emotions. Other times, we don't pay due attention and value to them. Our strategies may be inappropriate and ineffective or counterproductive in regulating the intensity or duration of what we feel.

Especially when experiencing intense emotions such as sadness, anxiety, anger, or fear, which can be perceived as uncontrolled and interfere with our normal social and psychological functioning.

Identifying, knowing, and improving our emotional competencies will help us manage our emotional world better, relate better with others, facilitate the achievement of our goals and objectives, and ultimately advance our well-being and personal growth.

Self-reflection: 3 questions about your emotional competencies

I propose three questions to start this interesting path towards your self-knowledge and expand the foundations of your emotional skills.

Use some everyday emotional reactions to increase your self-awareness:

- Identify what situation or event activated you. What was your emotional state like? How do you think you would react if you were cheerful, happy? What if you were mad or angry?
- Try to describe your thoughts and bodily sensations.
- If you thought differently, what would your emotional reaction be?

How do you change your negative emotions?

- Are you distracted, or do you think differently about what is affecting you?
- Do you focus on the positives?
- Are you trying to find solutions within your reach?
- Do you share your feelings with someone you trust?

Your communication with the people around you?

- Do they facilitate mutual understanding?
- Can they convey your emotions and opinions easily?
- Do they get you to understand other people's perspectives on disagreements?

Remember that this section's content is information. Even though it is scientific and rigorous and prepared by a team of experts, it has a formative, educational, or informative nature. It cannot be used or interpreted as a psychological or medical diagnosis. In health, specialists and accredited professionals are fundamental, who will always value each person's characteristics.

The global stigma around mental health

In recent times, more importance has been given to the disease of physical symptoms, but not so much to mental health, despite the WHO defining health as the complete state of physical, mental, and social well-being, and not only the absence of conditions or diseases.

We can go back to the end of the 1st century and the beginning of the 2nd century when the Roman author Juvenal wrote this Latin quote belonging to his satires "Mens sana in corpore sana." Something that we can interpret as the need for a healthy mind for a vitally important balance.

Canadian sociologist Erving Goffman is the author of a work entitled "Stigma," in which he defined stigma as the process in which the reaction of others spoils the "normal identity," recognizing the experience of mental illness as a form of stigma, it occurs in a wide variety of socio-political contexts in many parts of the world.

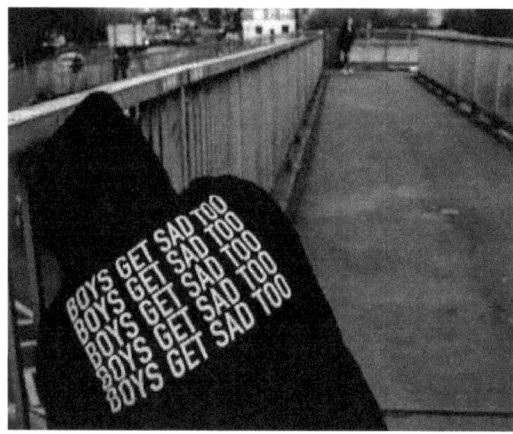

To address the stigma caused by mental illness, we must explain that it is a mental illness. Mental illness or disorder can be defined as an emotional, cognitive, or behavioral alteration in which basic psychological processes such as emotion, behavior, or learning are affected.

There are many mental diseases and disorders, including schizophrenia and psychotic disorders, mood disorders, anxiety disorders, dissociative disorders, personality disorders, adjustment disorders, bipolar disorder, somatoform disorders, and factitious disorders.

Mental illness is a great stigma in our society and especially in the developed world of the northern hemisphere. After an interview with a specialist in the field, and in which he dictates his diagnosis, the patient already lives with that stigma, the stigma of being seen differently from the rest of society, not fitting in, living socially isolated, and learn to live with a disease that often occurs chronically, with its consequent relapses and outbreaks.

Many people who have a mental disorder avoid talking about it to avoid social rejection. This link shows a video in which various patients tell about their experience with the disease and the difficulties they have had throughout his illness.

Most of society views these patients in derogatory terms, calling them 'crazy,' along with the belief that the mentally ill must be admitted to a psychiatric hospital.

According to the World Health Organization, one in four people will have a mental disorder in their lifetime, and by 2020 depression will be the second leading cause of disability in the world after coronary heart disease. Especially in the developed countries and the most robust economies of the northern hemisphere.

People with chronic mental illness have numerous rejection experiences, especially in the workplace, in social relationships, and in groups of friends: 44% claim to have had experiences of discrimination in the workplace, 43% in relationships with friends, and 32% with neighbors or their environment.

Some measures for the prevention of mental illnesses can be: regarding food, the consumption of vitamin B and DHA is recommended, which is a fatty acid that is part of Omega-3 and can be found in fish such as salmon or also in walnuts, almonds and peanuts; About exercise, it is recommended to carry out physical activities, thus allowing correct blood circulation in the cerebral vessels, optimizing mental function; In addition to exercise, intellectual activities such as reading and memory games are recommended.

I conclude with a phrase from the writer Ray Bradbury that says, "Madness is relative. It depends on who has whom locked in which cage". It is not a cause of infamy to suffer from a mental illness. The true infamy is not to be tolerant of those people who have a mental disorder. Usually, we talk about mental problems at a medical level: causes, symptoms, diagnoses, medications. Figures: how much of the population does it affect, what sex with the highest prevalence. However, this is never discussed, the taboo in our societies despite being something of such a high prevalence.

I doubt many people do not have close people with eating disorders, anxiety disorders, depression, etc. And it is very complicated because it is more, we have never been taught to learn to treat or help people with these types of problems, when what they need most is emotional support, to stop feeling like "strange creatures" and to feel integrated into a social circle.

On the other hand, the problems of depression are so much the order of the day and that everyone pretends not to know. Or if they know someone in this state, their contribution is to "dress up and paint yourself, and go for a walk," as if the person is unwell of their own free will.

Really, and unfortunately, today there is still this prejudice about people who we consider out of the "normal." Instead of listening to them and trying to help, we ignore them, turn our backs, mock and even make impediments so that they can develop a normal life. It is necessary to make known normally mental disorders, the people who suffer from them, and their internal struggle. With this, we will achieve its normalization in society. It is more important, in the health personnel who must support people with any type of physical or mental disorder contributing to their recovery. Still, we must apply it both to our work environment and in our daily lives.

Chapter 2: When the nights are blue and there's no meaning to it

We live in a culture that fosters wellness. We know what to eat, how many minutes to play sports and we spend hours staying relaxed to live better. But we have an Achilles heel: anxiety. According to the Anxiety and Depression Association of America, anxiety is the most common mental health problem, affecting more than 40 million adults across the United States.

However, anxiety is a natural protection mechanism, a psychological alert system that anticipates possible threats to avoid future problems. It is a state of restlessness, which **involves fear and stress at the same time when danger is not present**.

It's just an idea that springs up in your mind and creates the necessary stress to resolve your concerns before it's too late. Sometimes we have general anxiety that is not associated with any specific situation. It is nonspecific anxiety. Other times we know very well its origin: it is the specific one.

In both cases, it produces lightheadedness, nervousness, rapid heartbeat, sweating, tremors, choking, chest tightness, nausea, abdominal discomfort, dizziness, tingling (paresthesia), chills or flushing, fear of losing control, going crazy or dying, which produces isolation behaviors.

They are unpleasant enough sensations that we are often more afraid of anxiety itself than of the problem we are trying to solve: it is the fear of fear. If it is a normal emotion, why is it causing so much suffering and has it become an epidemic? Much of our education is based on being scared. According to Noam Chomsky, we live in the "**culture of fear**", a term to define the process by which this feeling is disseminated through the media, political speeches, etc. and that influences people's behavior.

Also, we have developed a phobia of uncertainty. We have a mania for the control that, paraphrasing Giorgio Nardone, ends up leading us to the abyss of uncontrolled.

The stress response activates **adrenaline** and **norepinephrine first**. The former increases the heart, and respiratory rate oxygenates the blood and increases blood pressure. The latter increases the capacity for analysis and motor coordination.

Then, the secretion of cortisol is activated, which favors the creation of circulating glucose, ensuring food for the brain (neurons eat glucose). It favors the mobilization of fat deposits so that the muscles move towards flight or fight. The persistence of this hormone can be very harmful. The systems that can be damaged by the anxiety response and stress are:

- Immune (allergies)
- Genetic (modifications in chromosomes)
- Neurological (headaches, memory loss, dizziness)
- Digestive (abdominal pain, gastritis, diarrhea and constipation)
- Cardiovascular (tachycardia, hypertension, palpitations)
- Respiratory (increased respiratory rate, cough, rhinitis)
- Cutaneous (sweating, tingling, eczema, alopecia)
- Genitourinary (frequent urination, premature ejaculation, impotence and frigidity)

Can we die? No, directly, but it involves physical wear and tear that favors these diseases.

Guilt trips

What is the origin of this discomfort that makes anxiety so little functional? This question has only one answer: your thoughts, according to cognitive psychology.

These produce distortions when it comes to orienting yourself in the world. They are the glasses that each one wears to look at reality. Which is yours?

- Pessimism: Tendency to focus on the problem without being able to see the solutions
- Generalization: Thoughts are always generalized
- Negative thinking: The focus is on the negative aspects, and the positive aspects are forgotten or disqualified
- Catastrophism: Seeing the negative aspects of an excessive and exaggerated way
- Reading the thought: They think they know what others are thinking and their hidden cynical motives
- Guessing the future: Tendency to anticipate that things will go wrong
- Comparison: Measure yourself against others to always end up losing and feeling inferior
- Exaggeration: If someone makes a mistake once they become clumsy or if one thing goes wrong they are called a failure in all areas
- Guilt: Feeling that the unpleasant circumstances that happen are always related to oneself
- Perfectionism: Making demands on others, on yourself or on how things should be

The feeling of vulnerability

What makes us vulnerable to anxiety problems? Emotional education plays a vital role in managing these types of thoughts. Also, there is a hereditary predisposition to suffer it. If your family has a history of anxiety disorders, you will be 45% more likely to suffer from them.

They influence, in turn, personality traits. The factors that lead to threatening interpretations are neuroticism (tendency to experience situations as unpleasant); the high sensitivity; introversion or tendency to over-excitement.

According to a study conducted at the University of Cambridge, the incidence of anxiety disorders skyrockets among **people who have not reached 35 years** of **age**, many of them are still students, an activity that increases anxiety.

Women are twice as likely to suffer from these disorders associated with family factors. For men, they are linked to economic and labor aspects. Children and adolescents suffer them linked to their evolutionary development, in **babies of eight or nine months** due to the need for contact.

At one or two years, separation anxiety is common, especially from the mother. **Between three and six years** is the adaptation to school and, after seven, meet the expectations of adults.

In **adolescence,** concerns revolve around self-image, group acceptance, and the future. Children show anxiety with somatic disorders ("my gut hurts") and phobias (fear of wasps, for example) and adolescents with obsessive disorders.

Anxiety in the elderly manifests itself with the deterioration of intellectual faculties (executive function, processing speed, memory and attention). Specialized help is needed when:

- Alterations in the person's family, work and social life;
- There is a risk to the physical and psychological integrity of oneself or of others;
- When symptoms persist for at least a month;
- The concern about the possibility of having more crises appears.

The modification of limiting beliefs by functional thoughts and interoceptive exposure (exposure to feared bodily sensations) works. For example, if you fear tachycardia, go up and downstairs and then calm yourself with relaxation or breathing techniques.

With systematic desensitization, the feared situation is gradually faced, first in the company and driving the distance until facing it directly. "Fear is my most faithful companion, it has never tricked me into going with another," says Woody Allen. However, we cannot allow ourselves to be manipulated by limiting thoughts and learn to manage them so that they do not block our life.

What is it like to live with anxiety? The story of a man and a woman

My dear friend Thomas (33 years old) recalls that he does not remember her life without anxiety. At just five years old, he began to feel extreme anguish when he stayed with a caregiver and suffered a seizure.

"At first, I did not know how to name what was happening. I called it being afraid, but I was afraid of many things," he explains.

With the support of different psychologists, he learned what was happening to him: he had anxiety. Identifying it and coping with professional help have taught him that, although "he will always be an anxious person", he can learn to live with this emotion.

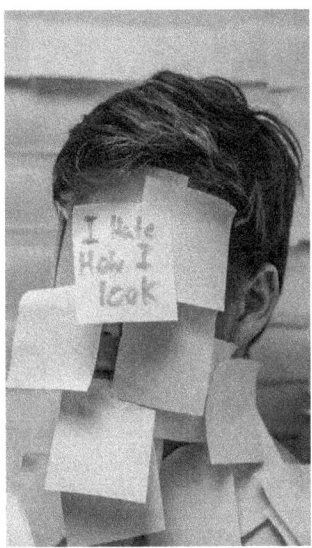

Anxiety is an innate adaptive capacity that is good; it prepares our body to face real danger and makes us able to flee from that danger more efficiently. However, as Thomas explains, when one suffers from an anxiety disorder "that fear seriously interferes in some important area of our life and becomes disabling."

If we look at the figures by gender, women who suffer from it almost double those of men. The symptoms of this disorder usually manifest in an alteration of the nervous system that produces hyperventilation, tachycardia and even dizziness.

According to the youth barometer of life and health, carried out by the Foundation for Help against Drug Addiction and the Mutua Madrileña Foundation, only half of the young people who feel symptoms of mental disorders go to a specialist.

Most cases of anxiety and depression begin in childhood and adolescence. By the time the patient demands care, more than ten years have passed, and they come to a consultation without having received any type of medical help.

However, with work and time, it can be minimized. From Thomas' experience, the key is that the person who suffers it "goes to a psychologist who teaches management and control strategies." Psychological treatment helps and does cure an anxiety disorder because it teaches you to manage it. And he adds: "More than controlling anxiety, you have to identify it, understand it and then regulate it."

I spoke to five more people who have learned to cope with their anxiety. Many of them began in childhood and adolescence, and all have been learning to handle it for years.

Helena García, 20 years old (Chicago)

"I have always suffered from anxiety. Since I was very little, I have felt nervous, very insecure, but I had not given it a name. I remember that in elementary school, I had problems to relate because I always thought about what they would think of me and that it generated a discomfort inside that gave me many problems.

"At the slightest feeling that something could go wrong I would start thinking about it and, after going all day at a thousand an hour in my head, I would go to bed and could not sleep. In high school, I remember three or four times that the next day I had an exam, and I could not go from the anxiety I had inside. I hadn't been able to stop crying all night, and I hadn't slept at all.

"Not sleeping started to become something that happened to me very often and my mother, who stayed up with me all night, told me one day that I couldn't go on like this and took me to the psychologist. By then, I was about 12 years old. Many people do not like to name their problems, but it helped me, because I knew something was wrong with me but not what it was. I saw that the source of my anxiety was my parents' relationship. As they were not well, I felt very lost, and that generated a lot of insecurities in me until I ended up exploding.

"When I was 14 years old, I had the occasional anxiety attack because everything came together: my parents ended up divorcing and it added to what I already had inside and to be in my teens. But at that age, I started with the medication and little by little. It got better. Some people believe that taking a pill is all right, but that is not the case. Medication without self-knowledge and without working on your emotions is useless. What I have improved since I started therapy until now is a world.

"Whenever I talk to people who have some kind of problem I tell them to go and ask for help. Although anxiety I don't think will go away (it is something that is part of my character) today I can say that you can control it and learn to live with it. But you always have to ask for help. It is useless if you keep it inside."

Caroline Armstrong, 27 years old (Denver)

"I started having generalized anxiety disorder when I was 20 years old. It was 2011, and I had just started a career in Gender Studies. Without really understanding the situation, I was walking down the street, and I felt sad and nervous. For example, on the subway, if I stopped between two stations, I would turn white and have a tachycardia. I felt paralyzed and even stopped riding on it. But then he couldn't put a name to something he didn't know."

Caroline began to have anxiety when she was 20 years old.

"My mother decided to take me to a psychologist when she saw me like this. While in consultation, I realized that I suffered from anxiety about a lot of things. I had a difficult adolescence, I am a very self-demanding person, and in high school, I felt that I had to comply with everything. She had to be the perfect partner, and if she wasn't, it frustrated me. I ended up paying for it with food, and I got really fat.

"In the end, anxiety is like the tip of the iceberg of what is happening to you. There are internal things that you have to solve. Going to therapy, I realized that I had the baggage of adolescence with complexes and that I felt insecure with myself.

"I spent four years with the psychologist; Four years that were hard, but also beautiful because they made me learn about my life, boost my self-esteem and feel more empowered. The person who started has nothing to do with who I am now. In your day to day affairs, you continue to have anxiety or that predisposition, but when you see it as a threat, you apply the techniques you have learned."

Albert Miller II, 45 years old (New York)

"When I was 36 years old, I began to notice sensations in myself that I didn't know how to interpret. My father had died two years before, and that setback that I experienced I think made me more vulnerable. I spent a long time feeling dizzy, sleeping poorly and having the impression that everything I did at work was beyond me. I went to the emergency room for this feeling of dizziness (which made me even stop riding my bike) where they told me that I had nothing and that what I had to do was relax. But one day, I got up and exploded.

"I started crying like a child and told my wife that I felt unable to go to work. I took the step and took my first anxiety leave. I joined my job as Senior IT Manager after four months on the job and, after 11 years with the company, I was fired the same day I returned."

Albert realized that he was doing a job that he did not like.

"So I decided with my wife that the first three months of my son's life (who was born after the layoff) I would live with him at home. And those three months turned into three years. It was the perfect excuse to escape the subject and avoid the scenario where it had started: the world of work.

"I was interspersing other jobs, but for four and a half years it was all very intermittent because I kept giving up due to anxiety and they ended up firing me. But I found a psychologist who allowed me to understand how it affected me in my day to day life. It was here when I began to 'dominate' it, and little by little, it disappeared. After this, I realized that I was doing a job that I did not like, and after going against the current for so long, my body was manifesting it in this way.

"For a year and a half I have changed my life, I have stopped working as a computer scientist and have started volunteering in associations related to mental health. This has been somewhat therapeutic and, although I have sacrificed the purchasing power and advantages that my previous job offered me, the feeling I have is completely different. I have the reins of my life again. I wish the changes were not traumatic and with suffering involved, but in my case, it has been a change with which I have come out winning."

Pamela Wright Thompson, 33 years old (Los Angeles)

"I don't remember my life without anxiety. I started having it from a very young age. When I was five years old, I remember that I had a panic attack because my parents and my brothers went rafting to a river and I was left alone with a caretaker from the hotel where we were.

"At that time, I called it 'being afraid,' and I was afraid of many things. My parents found out and started taking me to the psychologist. Although she tells it like that, she was a happy girl, but she had many fears. I had a good time in high school, but when I got to college, everything started to get worse. I broke up with my partner. My family went through a process of seizure of our house... It was all very stressful.

"Also, a friend of mine committed suicide, and I started having obsessive thoughts that I was scared to kill myself too. I didn't want to, of course, but the very thought of it terrified me. From the anxiety that these thoughts produced in me, I even saw the crooked floor, and I found myself dizzy all the time. It was constant anxiety.

"I went back to the psychologist, and he said it was an 'impulse phobia' and that he was afraid of getting out of control. Those thoughts were intrusive, I didn't choose them, but they meant absolutely nothing: thinking about suicide did not mean that I was going to commit suicide, only that I had focused my stress on that idea.

"To this was added that in my environment, my anxiety was not well seen. People don't understand what anxiety entails, and this misunderstanding made me suffer much more than necessary. But with the psychologist, it went so well that I began to control it. I was 23 years old, and I started a radio master's degree, I started living alone.

"Little by little, I was coming out of that dark time of obsessions. I've never had a period of such anxiety like that again. Now I control it more, but it still affects me. I've always been anxious, and I realize it's one thing I'll always have. "

How to control anxiety?

Anxiety is a state of activation of the nervous system that is oriented towards the anticipation of danger, whether real or imagined. Being something so general, it has a physiological and a psychological aspect: in the first, there are phenomena such as tremors, sweating and acceleration of the pulse, and in the second there are phenomena such as the emotion of fear, the desire to avoid a stimulus aversive, and difficulties in controlling emotional responses to a situation.

Maintain regular routines

It is very important to be able to continue with the day to day routine, and that anxiety does not "gain ground". This means that the person must make an effort to maintain their activities and try not to avoid those situations that generate anxiety.

For example, if after the treatment you have managed to take the subway to go to work, even if it still generates a little anxiety, it is very important to continue practicing this situation to make the anxiety decrease

Play sports and doing exercise

Regular physical activity is advisable for almost everyone, and people with an anxiety disorder are no exception. Some scientific studies conclude that physical exercise (regular and moderate intensity) can help reduce and relieve anxiety symptoms.

Have good eating and sleeping habits

Maintaining proper eating and sleeping habits is essential to maintaining a healthy lifestyle. Sleeping for fewer hours than is recommended in a sustained way can cause irritability or stress, an aspect that can negatively affect anxiety symptoms.

Do not take stimulants in excess

The use of stimulants such as coffee, in high amounts and for long periods, can increase anxiety levels.

Avoid intoxicants

Some people with anxiety disorders use certain substances (such as alcohol or cannabis) to reduce the discomfort caused by some anxiety symptoms. However, doing this does not make the symptoms disappear in the medium / long term and increases the risk of problems related to substance abuse.

Be active on a social level

A good social circle that allows you to be active with friends can be a good tool to combat depressive symptoms (sadness or excessive apathy) that some people with anxiety disorders may have.

Share discomfort with the immediate environment

Some people can benefit from sharing their discomfort with those around them or with support groups. It is important to feel relieved, as well as for people around you to help identify the first symptoms of a relapse, for example.

Comply with the treatment

Following treatment, guidelines are important to combat anxiety symptoms. There are people with an anxiety disorder who may need to take medication for long periods. In these cases, the person may lose motivation, thinks about stopping the treatment or gets tired of some side effects. It is very important to express these doubts or reluctance to the health team to assess the best treatment options.

Enter depression

Depression does not always manifest it in the same way. Nor does it only imply a sad person who does not stop crying. There are many realities, and all of them deserve to be attended with the utmost professionalism and affection. Sufferers of depression are not always understood by society.

What is depression? Often this question has an easy answer when associating the word depression to the feeling of "being sad" or "having little desire to do anything".

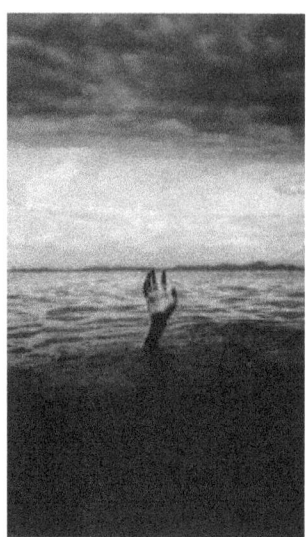

Although in reality, these feelings are unpleasant. Sharing company with others suffering from depression would be just the tip of the iceberg of a disease that is increasingly present in our daily lives and with figures on the rise over the next few years.

Thus, a recent WHO estimate reveals that by 2020 of all diseases, depression will be the second most widespread in the world. As an additional characteristic that makes this disease especially dangerous and that is in the focus of mental health, is the presence of self-destructive behaviors in people who suffer from it.

Ultimately, to try to address depression, we cannot assume that this disease is only caused by "a handful of symptoms", such as feelings of sadness or dejection, not even as a syndrome (set of symptoms), such as sadness, anxiety, insomnia, etc.

It should be classified as a disorder, where this set of symptoms would be encompassed in a whole, which would affect the person who suffers from it in all its context, negatively influencing their family, partner, socially, in performance at work or study, in their health and the absence of daily activities in general.

What is the origin of depression?

Is there any cause that can explain its appearance? Much has been written about different factors or events that promote depression. Although these factors are not exclusive of other variables that may predispose to increase the appearance of the disease or prevent it from appearing, it is possible to speak of genetic or biochemical factors as a fundamental cause.

Regarding specific stressful situations that favor the appearance of depression, there are those situations of loss or grief, current or past traumatic situations and stressful factors in the life of this person, although as indicated above, the appearance or not of the disease, is the combination of such events with other biological and psychological factors,

Depression being, therefore a disorder, **how will it affect a person who suffers from it?** To understand the answer to this question, a support point must be established in the Beck (1973) model, which does not speak of a series of ad hoc characteristics, but the combination of the present symptoms, together with the evolution of these long-term symptoms, as well as the intensity of them.

Taking into account how these symptoms can evolve, a series of responses appear in people with the disorder:

- **Physiological/emotional responses:** Appearance of sadness, irritability, anxiety, sleep disturbances (excess or deficiency), loss of appetite, decreased sexual desire, the appearance of pain in the body's joints (knees, arms, jaw)
- **Cognitive responses**: Desire to escape, erroneous thoughts that increase the perception of disability of the person suffering from the disease, thoughts of guilt for not being able to get out of the situation, difficulty in making decisions, negative self-regard, negative world, denial of the future, attention difficulties, memory problems, suicidal ideas, passivity, difficulty in social relationships, dependence, loss of motivation and ability to enjoy and seek happiness.
- **Motor responses:** Difficulties falling asleep, waking up very early, agitation, psychomotor inhibition, crying.

These three responses are combined, forming a characteristic style of behavior in these people that are included in the famous "three A's."

- **Abulia:** Decreased interest and the ability to obtain pleasure in the activities that the person performs.
- **Apathy:** Feeling of lack of energy that leads these people to stop performing daily activities, because they find these activities especially heavy or tired.
- **Anhedonia:** Reduction of activities that the person suffering from the disorder found rewarding before the onset of the disease. The person stops going out with friends, attending family gatherings, doing sports or leisure activities in general, because they find their state of mind "stiff", not perceiving the happiness they used to find in such activities.

These styles of behavior make these people choose to be in bed or sitting in an armchair without the desire to actively assume any type of behavior, with feelings of hopelessness along with feelings of anxiety, and hyperactivity.

The depressed person sees their desire to continue with the usual activities altered, and the feeling of hopelessness immobilizes them to express their feelings, which ends up making it difficult for other members of a family or friends of this person to understand the seriousness of their state.

Depression is considered one of the most dangerous mental disorders that exist. As mentioned above, the functional state of the person who suffers from it is very deteriorated, but why consider dangerous a disorder that only affects the daily functioning of a person?

Indeed, if we let ourselves be carried away by the symptoms and signs of this disease, it does not seem that it is a serious disorder. However, let's analyze the self-destructive and hopeless thoughts of those who suffer it. It is not difficult for us to see the final solution that someone who spends many hours bedridden, analyzing all the characteristics of their life negatively, blaming themselves and not seeing a clear solution to their problems.

If, as stated in the previous point, depression is so serious, how is it possible that it is not stopped with useful prevention or intervention programs?

The answer at this point is clear, not because of financing problems or because there are no useful prevention programs, the answer to this question simply involves the behavior of the person who suffers from it. Thus, when it comes to diagnosing and treating the pathology, there are three types of possible cases:

- People who go to their primary care doctor, where they detect the depressive picture and an appropriate pharmacological and psychological treatment is established
- Those who go early to the primary care doctor, but depression is not detected. This can occur because the person does not want to admit that he or she has a mental disorder and derives attention to the organic symptoms, not paying attention to other signs or mental processes that the patient decides to omit or the doctor does not ask.
- Finally, those people who decide not to go to the primary care doctor, making their disorder chronic.

Which of these three types of cases occurs most often?

The first case, although it would be the most appropriate, is the least frequent. The second of the three cases, although present, is no longer so present, since there are currently very competent programs in the global healthcare system that have improved the diagnosis of the disease.

As for the last case, unfortunately, it is the most frequent. Since people with depression, omit from their family and friends the seriousness of their thoughts or feelings, leaving only their motor behavior evident, passing their friends or family to perceive them as a "lazy", "crybaby" or "exaggerated" person who spends all day lying down without doing anything, lamenting his sadness, in such a way that they avoid going to a specialist.

This increases the chances of the disorder to manifest further. And therefore, the severity and probability of self-injurious behaviors, the most serious being suicide. According to WHO data, a person with depression is 30 times more likely to threaten his life than any other person.

This inability to request help has become the most urgent problem in public health, since in most cases, when people with depression go to primary care, they do so because other symptoms that afflict these people are observed, in greater case anxiety or panic attacks.

As if that were not enough, it is currently estimated that this mood disorder is among the most prevalent psychiatric conditions. Thus epidemiological data suggest that 17% of the population reported having experienced depression at some point in their life; that is, at least once a day, primary care physicians treat a person with depression.

If this disorder has the World Health Organization in check, **what are the expectations for treatment or cure?**

Undoubtedly, drug treatment with antidepressants is the most widely used and fundamental treatment to tackle the problem in the short-medium term. However, it has been proven that in the long term, the possibility that the disorder may appear is greater.

Then a combined treatment is exercised with some type of psychological therapy.

Although cognitive-behavioral therapy is the one that has been used the most for its effectiveness and many years of experience, as well as the research behind it, new therapies are currently appearing that are showing even better results. These are the third generation behavioral therapy or ACT, Cognitive-Analytical therapy and EMDR therapy.

In any case, it is the combined pharmacological and psychological treatment that has the best results not only in the first phases of treatment but also in the prevention of relapses.

The reasons and symptoms are different according to gender and are linked to social constructions.

You cannot cry because crying does not come from you. Sometimes you don't want to talk because you don't know what to say. This is how Rodrigo Vera, a 28-year-old communication specialist, defines depression. For him, to suffer, it is to carry inside the biggest hole.

Depression is a mental disorder that is different from the usual mood swings. Depressive episodes can be classified as mild, moderate or severe. At least one in five people will have a depressive episode before reaching the age of 75.

Rodrigo suffers from chronic depression. However, it is estimated that the number could be higher due to how complex it is to identify the disorder. Although in many cases depression is described as a "deep nostalgic mood", he speaks of life in depression as "unpleasant", like a void that is not filled with music, food, colors, reading or loved ones.

"I identify myself among people who appear to be fine, but who suddenly enter into crises that seem to come out of nowhere. And on other occasions I don't identify with any of the symptoms that you see on the subway posters about depression and suicides," Rodrigo explains in one of our exclusive conversations for this chapter.

Unlike sadness, depression is a condition that has physical and cognitive symptoms. The two main ones are feeling sad most days of the week with a duration of at least two weeks and anhedonia, which is the loss of will, desire, interest or pleasure for things that previously did cause it.

There are physical symptoms such as insomnia or sleeping too much, increased or decreased appetite, memory problems or to maintain long periods of attention, which are related to forgetfulness, confusion and poor school or work performance.

Having ups and downs in a society like the current one is the norm, it would be strange if we didn't have them. However, it emphasizes the importance of not confusing between transitory states, which all people go through, and the diagnosis of depression.

Depression in women

"One of the problems I had with my mother was getting her to accept that something was wrong with me. For her, going to the psychologist was an exaggeration, a way of seeking care. And if we were talking about a psychiatrist, even worse," says 26-year-old Teresa Robles.

She wants both her mother and her friends to understand that feeling like this is not her decision and that having depression does not mean "being sad all the time". For Tere, living with depression has been a journey in which she has understood that there is nothing wrong with feeling this way, but that at the same time it is something to fight to avoid being a prisoner of the disease.

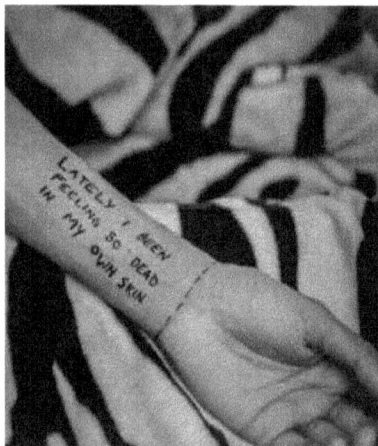

Clara Fleiz Bautista, from the "Ramón de la Fuente Muñiz" National Institute of Psychiatry, explains that for every two women with depression, one man suffers from it. This prevalence of the disorder is mainly due to gender stereotypes that generate anguish or tension for women.

Frequently, the mandates of motherhood, femininity related to aesthetics and gender violence, are associated with the depression experienced by women, the researcher Lucía Ciccia also agrees. "The symptoms to which depression is associated are linked to feelings, and that is something that is deeply associated with the feminine".

According to the specialist, the fact that the symptoms are "feminized" is because women express sadness more easily with crying or seeking medical attention. At the same time, men tend to express depression through irritability or anger.

The psychologist by the UAM, specialized in care for women survivors of gender violence, Martha Viniegra, estimates that depression in women is diagnosed three times more frequently than in men.

"Masculinity prevents you from going to the doctor until there is a crisis. Men are educated to seek success, be assertive and self-confident, but women are not".

On the other hand, men register a greater consumption of substances such as alcohol or drugs, often to "mask a psychiatric problem such as depression or anxiety and to substitute medical attention." Another revealing fact is that unsuccessful suicide attempts are more common in women, while men do tend to commit suicide.

When Tere was prescribed medications to treat the depression and anxiety that she was diagnosed with, her mother objected to her taking them, not believing what was happening to her and thinking that she was going to become dependent on them.

Adults with depressive episodes or with chronic depression usually undergo treatment that lasts 9 to 12 months, but it does not apply to all types of depression.

A parameter for prescribing medications to a person with severe depression is when they have a complete loss of sleep or, on the contrary, they sleep for days. Besides, they are absent from work or school and do not see their loved ones as often as before.

Patients often believe that they will not be well again without the help of medications or that they will need other treatments to feel well. It is as if the person with diabetes says he cannot depend on his medicine. It is a deficiency that the body has and must be resolved with some treatment or therapy.

The specialist likes the comparison between diabetes and depression, because just as the diabetic patient is not only treated with medication, those with depression must also do the "diet and exercise" that diabetic patients would do. In this case, they are psychotherapies.

Talk about depression

Many people avoid talking about depression or any mental health topic because they are topics that "carry a negative charge, compared to success, that is painted with a smile." The world abounds with examples of people who are considered successful (with work, family and pleasures) and despite that feel sad.

In the world, 300 million people suffer from depression, a figure equivalent to the entire population of Indonesia. Despite being such a common disease, there are taboos around it that must be eliminated to face it as the serious public health problem that it is.

"I think that the people closest to me think that my problem is not a problem and that is something dangerous because when I fall into those states of sadness, I feel deeply alone and responsible. For me, that is the biggest dilemma of depression," shared Rodrigo.

Dr Lucía Ciccia defines depression as a social epidemic that does not have viral contagion but feeds on the ease with which it is diagnosed, and antidepressants are presented, instead of pointing out the structural factors that generate this health problem.

"Generating social conditions in which you can move in a way that makes you feel better is much more difficult than taking a pill. Although a pill is necessary as a palliative in extreme cases, it should not be the easy medicine or the solution", says the CIEG researcher.

Movies that accurately depict mental illnesses

Taboos surround mental illnesses, and it is difficult to understand the situation of the people who suffer from them. Currently, we live in a world where culture is influenced by film and television. A great option to help society understand, empathize and understand.

Any movie offers a psychological reading of its characters and their way of thinking. It is very important to find characters with whom we feel identified. For this reason, it is just as important that people who suffer from some type of mental illness or those who care for a dependent person feel identified with certain cinematographic characters.

Personality disorders, schizophrenia, Alzheimer's and many more pathologies are reflected in the cinema. However, most of the time, the visibility they give to mental illnesses is usually unrealistic and even dangerous.

The mentally ill are often depicted as delusional murderers or villains; this is a gross misrepresentation of reality. For this reason, I have numbered the films that realistically present mental illnesses, to understand the people who suffer from these mental illnesses.

The best mental illness movies to understand:

Always Alice (2014)

It is a film that tries to bring us closer to the feelings of those who have Alzheimer's and their families.

Alice is proud of the life that has taken her so much effort to build. At 50, she is a professor of psychology at Harvard and a world-renowned linguist expert, with three grown children and a successful husband.

One day, she begins to feel disoriented, and a tragic diagnosis changes her entire life, influencing her relationships with her family and with the entire world. Alzheimer's has come to mind.

Love and other drugs (2011)

Maggie is a girl who will not allow anything or anyone to tie her up in her day to day life. Everything changes when you find your ideal partner. Jamie is an attractive 30-year-old man who does not hesitate to use his charm on girls and who lives in the ambitious world of pharmaceutical sales.

What at first starts as a relationship based on sex and ease, ends up becoming a relationship full of obstacles. Jaime's great dedication to his work is a great obstacle, but the worst is the secret that Maggie keeps; suffers from a degenerative disease, Parkinson's.

Melancholy (2011)

This film paints a very realistic picture of how the world collapses every day for people who suffer from depression, although the next day they may see everything better.

Justine sabotages her wedding night and falls into an almost catatonic depression. You cannot bathe or eat without having an ash taste in your mouth. Each member of her family represents a trait of humanity that contributes to Justine's state of mind.

Black Swan (2010)

Black Swan is based on metaphor to achieve perfection, whatever the price to achieve it.

Nina, a brilliant dancer from New York, lives completely absorbed by dance. She has an eating disorder as well as chronic hallucinations.

Many professionals in the world of dance suffer from eating disorders. The anorexia nervosa is one of the most common eating disorders and is considered the deadliest mental illness today.

The Machinist (2004)

The driver shows a very real vision of what it is like to suffer from chronic insomnia.

The protagonist of this film, Trevor, suffers from an extreme case of insomnia. This affects your day-to-day life and brings you numerous problems.

Trevor begins to hallucinate while at work and leaves his colleagues in dangerous situations without realizing it. For this, they blame him for several incidents and make his life impossible.

He ends up paranoid, fighting with everyone and constantly seeing hallucinations. *Will he be able to recover?*

Noa's Diary (2004)

The film is based on a love story told through Noa's diary, which he reads to his wife continuously. He hopes that his wife will remember what she had experienced with him and so he can enjoy a few seconds of lucidity with his wife since she has Alzheimer's.

Big Fish (2003)

A nice story of a boy with his father. William does not have a good relationship with his father Albert. Still, after learning that he is terminally ill, he returns to his side: Albert has a schizotypal personality disorder and spends the day telling his endless stories from his youth.

On this occasion, William will try to find out things that will allow him to know his father better. To do this, you must distinguish between reality and fantasy.

A Wonderful Mind (2001)

It is a biographical drama of the famous mathematician John Nah. The story is based on John's life, as he slowly develops paranoid schizophrenia.

The film gives an insight into how to learn to live with schizophrenia and fight for all your dreams despite it.

Memento (2000)

"Memento" is a confusing and entertaining movie at the same time. It shows us two different versions of the same scene throughout the movie. In black and white, in color and with different timelines. This is for the public to put themselves in the shoes of Leonard, a character suffering from anterograde amnesia.

Anterograde amnesia is a memory disorder that prevents a person from creating new memories after the event that caused dementia.

Fight Club (1999)

In *"Fight Club"* we have two main characters: an unnamed narrator and Tyler.

Tyler is a pimp who makes soap; the narrator is dissatisfied with his life who suffers from a multiple personality disorder. The narrator turns into Tyler to make up for his lack of power and masculinity. It portrays the disease very well and is a legitimate representation of how intense this disorder can be.

Why therapy?

Although society evolves and accepts new cultures, new fashions, and new diseases, mental disorders remain an indecent subject; Many times the fact of attending a psychological consultation is strange for others, for which the acceptance of a mental illness for those who suffer from it, becomes much more complex. Not to mention that the suffering produces a cognitive deterioration reflected in distorted thoughts and irrational ideas, which become the daily lives of patients, taking away the tranquility of them and those around them.

In this sense, the vast majority of people who are diagnosed with a mental illness, their therapy begins with taking pharmacological medications (psychiatry), to stabilize the person from their altered state of consciousness; However, cognitive-behavioral therapy has proven to be an indispensable tool for obtaining more effective prognoses in treatments.

On the other hand, the diagnosis of a mental disorder includes significant changes in the life of the person suffering from it and of those around him, the transformations can range from eating behavior to creating a new social circle, forcing the patient to modify many areas of your life.

In this vein, it becomes clear that the impact of the diagnosis of any physical and mental illness generates various questions in the patient, such as: where does the disease come from? Why does it give? Cure? Why me? Which on occasions, tend to be answered inadequately or simply not answered, which causes patients who drop out of the treatments and constant relapses.

Among the treatments available for those who suffer from some type of mental disorder, psychoactive drugs and psychotherapy are considered, which have shown similar efficacy if we stick to the mere reduction of symptoms.

However, psychiatry has sometimes fallen short as a single treatment, which has promoted psychotherapy as a complement to the efficiency of the processes, is as well as recently the World Psychiatry magazine, one of the most renowned psychiatric publications at an international level, has shown the effectiveness of the interventions psychological disorders in the treatment of serious mental disorders, in the absence of new drugs that act effectively.

However, it continues to seem like a second option.

According to the Diagnostic and Statistical Manual (DSM) in its different versions, it conceptualizes mental disorder as "a syndrome or a behavioral or psychological pattern of clinical significance, which appears associated with discomfort, a disability or a significantly increased risk of dying or of suffering pain, disability or loss of freedom."

This manual makes categorization of types of mental disorders, which demand different methods and patient care, either with pharmacological and psychological treatments; the latter, the psychological model that best adapts to the DSM is the cognitive one (psychotherapy cognitive), which is based on the diagnostic criteria of this manual and proposes that "all mental disturbances have in COMMON a distortion of thought, which influences the mood and behavior of patients".

Thus, one of the treatments for mental disorders is psychotherapy, which is presented as a procedure where a professional in psychology uses techniques to help a person overcome their psychological difficulties, to achieve psychological well-being and the adaptation of the subject; in this, there are several approaches and intervention techniques, which allow the patient the most appropriate choice of his therapist.

In the case of psychotherapeutic support in the diagnosis of a mental illness, cognitive-behavioral therapy is presented as one of the first choice treatments, based on the principles, mechanisms and processes that govern abnormal behavior provided by other scientific disciplines of psychology, such as psychopathology, learning psychology, and cognitive psychology.

About the above, in 1998 the American Psychological Association, to evaluate the efficacy of psychological treatments, established the following criteria for measuring the effectiveness of therapies, if: "their efficacy is empirically supported by results of at least two intergroup experimental studies or 10 SINGLE-case experimental studies, which demonstrate that said therapy is superior to drug treatment, a psychological placebo or another alternative psychological treatment, or that it is equivalent to a well-established treatment ".

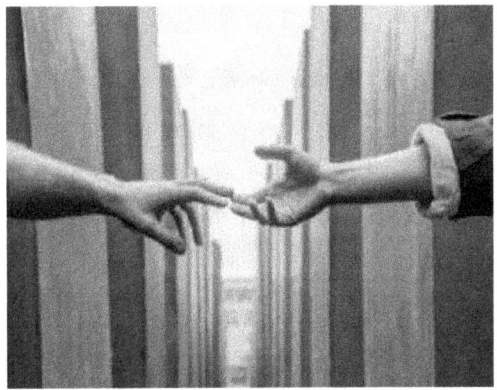

This is how this therapeutic approach is focused on problems and difficulties of the here and now, that is, it works directly on the irrational and the distorted in mental illness as its maintenance factors; for this, the main objective is the solution of the patient's problems, through behavioral, cognitive and emotional change. One of the key characteristics is that it lies in the subjective and behavioral connections of the beliefs, feelings and actions of the patient, regardless of whether these beliefs are based on reality.

Besides, these are two models with a wide research trajectory: cognitive and behavioral; the first focuses on the identification of mental schemes and processes, with which the patient interprets and gives a meaning about himself and the world; the second is based on external behavior, and the basic processes of learning; The union of these two approaches aims to modify the way people think, through strategies investigated in advance with case studies.

Some of the strategies are systematic desensitization, Ellis's rational emotional-behavioral therapy, Beck's cognitive therapy, among others. Mixed procedures, where work is done on the cognitive, affective aspect and behavioral, are the best since they encompass the whole person".

Likewise, what cognitive-behavioral psychotherapy seeks in the treatment of mental disorders is for the patient to show his interpretations about his disease, understand it and, above all, accept it, helping him to define goals and teaching him to apply techniques psychological that contribute to reducing the discomfort associated with the disorder.

It is important to note that in most medical treatments for mental illnesses, pharmacology plays a fundamental role for the stability and proper functioning of the subject, however, not all people have the ability to transform their lives and accept a disease.

But then, what happens if the medications do not clarify the thoughts, the way of seeing the world and the issues that patients present? It is there where the biological factor ceases to be the main one, and other factors such as sociocultural and psychological are included.

Psychotherapy is charged with power and becomes necessary in this process, to create awareness of the disease, for adherence to pharmacology, knowledge of its symptoms, early arrest of episodes, to help a patient to distinguish and recognize what affects him, encourage responsibility, self-care, the ability to choose and decide, evaluating and assuming the consequences that this implies.

Additionally, cognitive-behavioral psychotherapy offers psychoeducation for the families or caregivers of the patient, training them on the diagnosis and providing them with the tools to understand and manage the person who suffers from it. Also, they are given a guide on what factors can improve or worsen the prognosis, reducing the burden and stress of the family, achieving greater emotional stability.

Psychoeducational programs for family members aimed at increasing knowledge about mental illness and changing attitudes are USEFUL within the scope of family intervention, in reducing the risk of relapse in patients.

On the other hand, it is important for the effectiveness of the treatment, that between the therapist and the patient, a level of trust (rapport) is achieved that allows them to establish a transparent conversation, where the patient freely expresses their thoughts, without fear of feeling judged or rejected.

This connection enables the therapist to assume a leading role in the life and recovery of the person suffering from the diagnosis, "supported by the certainty that he has a knowledge and an attitude to put them in favor of the well-being of his patient, and as a consequence, the patient assumes a submissive and waiting position in front of the cure. For all that has been said, it is important to analyze the benefits that psychotherapy can have in the lives of patients, prioritizing it as a comprehensive treatment for them; However, the diagnosis of mental illnesses can be similar to a dental problem.

It can suffer like a toothache due to cavities, and this causes the person to attend their dentist, who immediately performs an oral cleaning, stabilizing the pain, also gives a series of recommendations, such as brushing their teeth three times a day and for greater care and efficiency the use of dental floss. Many patients are left with the first recommendation as it is the most used, and dental floss takes a back seat.

Similarly, in the diagnosis of mental disorders, they are generally made when the patient goes into crisis, he goes to a psychiatrist, who, like the dentist, tries to reduce the symptoms with medications, achieving mental stability immediately.

However, the psychiatrist makes a series of recommendations, among which is attendance at psychotherapy and support groups, which allow them to educate themselves about the disease; recommendation that is evaded by the patient, who, for the most part, prioritize the use only of drugs and omits attendance at psychotherapy, which produces less effective treatments.

It is necessary to increase the effective perspective compared to psychotherapy, because only a small proportion of patients suffering from mental disorders receive therapeutic support, even though this is valid and efficient, and can be used much more generalized. Thus, it is of great importance to encourage in the field of mental health, among medical professionals, psychiatrists and psychologists, that from their exercise, the treatment of disorders is complemented with psychotherapy, as a priority tool in education, control and acceptance of the patient in his diagnosis. So that the results are more successful and social, personal, emotional and physical benefits can be obtained that allow you to have a life with greater well-being.

Chapter 3: The Global Crisis of Mental Health

Mental health is described as a state of well-being in which people are conscious of their skills. It has to do with encouraging well-being, preventing mental illnesses and treating and rehabilitating individuals affected by these conditions.

Depression and anxiety disorders are prevalent mental health conditions that influence the ability to function and productivity. More than 300 million people, recognized as one of the major causes of disability, suffer from depression. More than 260 million people in the world have anxiety disorders at the same time.

In Latin America, the prevalence of psychiatric and neurological disorders over 12 months (or the number of cases during this period ranges between 18.7 and 24.2 percent; that of anxiety disorders, between 9.3 and 16.1 percent; that of affective disorders, between 7.0 and 8.7 percent; and that of psychoactive drug use disorders, between 3.6 percent and 5.3 percent.

According to the WHO Mental Health Action Plan, persons with major depression or schizophrenia are 40 to 60 percent more likely than the general population to die prematurely because of physical health conditions that are often not treated (e.g. cancers, cardiovascular disease, diabetes, and HIV infection) and suicide.

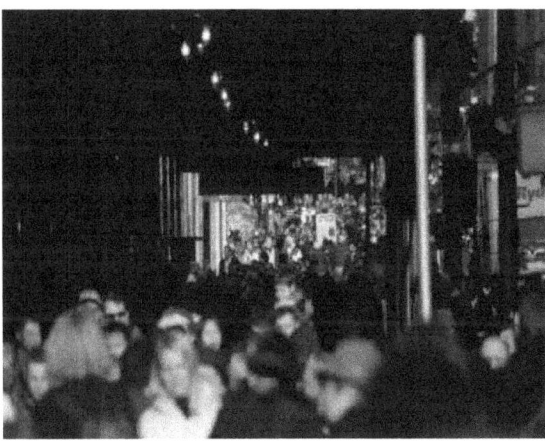

Equally wide are the economic effects of mental disorders such as depression or others. A World Economic Forum report estimated that between 2011 and 2030, the total global effects of mental illness in terms of economic losses would be $16.3 billion.

A brief history of mental illnesses

1906: At the XXXVII Southwest German Psychiatric Conference, the pathologist and psychiatrist Alois Alzheimer presented a specific cerebral cortex disease.

1949: Mental Health America launches efforts in the United States to commemorate Mental Health Month in May.

1996: publication of the work on the global burden of mental illness by the WHO and the Institute for Health Measurement and Evaluation.

2011: Publication by the WHO of the Intervention Guide for mental, neurological, and substance use disorders.

2012: The 65th World Health Assembly adopted resolution WHA65.4 on the global burden of mental disorders and the need for a comprehensive and coordinated response by the health and social sectors of the countries

2013: The World Health Assembly approved a comprehensive plan of action on mental health for 2013-2020.

2017: The World Health Assembly endorsed the Global Plan of Action on the Public Health Response to Dementia 2017-2025.

It is difficult to find a concept so diffuse and so used at the same time as that of mental health. The notion of mental health refers to a state or condition of the individual, to a field – conceptual and practical – within public health, to a series of psychiatric pathologies and psychosocial problems, even to a set of health and social initiatives.

Since the end of the Second World War and until today, mental health has acquired an extraordinary role, both at an academic and political level and in the daily life of Western societies. In 1946, the *Mental Health Association* was founded in London and, two years later, the First International Congress on Mental Health was held in the same city.

The World Health Organization, since its origins in 1948, has a Mental Health section. And in 1949, the *National Institute of Mental Health was created in the USA*. This reflects the interest in the great world powers' subject for decades, which, far from diminishing, grows every day.

It is not an exaggeration to say that we are experiencing a true mental health boom, although we do not always know what we are talking about.

In 1950, a WHO expert committee presented the first definition of mental health, clearly influenced by dynamic psychiatry. The three criteria proposed to define a mentally healthy person are:

- Achieving a satisfactory synthesis of one's instincts, potentially conflictive
- Establishing and maintaining harmonious relationships with others
- The possibility of modifying the physical and social environment.

It should be noted that we are in the difficult post-war years and that the term that is most repeated in this definition is "harmony." Shortly after, in 1958, the social psychologist Marie Jahoda published her famous systematization of positive mental health in the USA – created at the behest of the *Joint Commission on Mental Illness and Health* –, which has been widely disseminated, simplified, and which undoubtedly constitutes the most obvious reference of all subsequent definitions.

The criteria proposed by Jahoda are:

- Realistic self-concept, identity, and self-esteem,
- Search for growth and self-actualization
- Integration of oneself and the different experiences,
- Autonomy,
- Objective perception of the reality
- Mastery of the environment: adaptation and success to achieve goals

For decades, we have bodies of the highest level in charge of mental health, and with more or less official definitions. However, these descriptions, in addition to not being without criticism, are outweighed by the daily use of the notion of mental health.

And it is actually: "mental health is presented as a generic object, under which a dispersed set of discourses and practices on mental disorders, psychosocial problems, and well-being are sheltered"; discourses and practices that "obey the rationalities of the different approaches to health and disease in the field of public health, philosophy, psychology, anthropology, psychiatry, among others, and therefore, mental health conceptions depend on these approaches and the ideologies that underlie them" (Restrepo & Jaramillo: 2012, p. 203).

It is difficult to understand that kind of kaleidoscope that both mental health-oriented practices and the definitions of mental health constitute without delving into the disciplines and discourses that have contributed to creating this field.

Psychiatry, the different psychotherapies, and movements critical to psychological and psychiatric clinics, such as antipsychiatry, community psychology, and other movements closer to social medicine and even to political action.

In general, both in academic texts, public plans and policies, and health services, the expression "psychiatry and mental health" is used. The use of the conjunction indicates that we should not confuse both terms, fields, or disciplines, that psychiatry and mental health are two issues that go together, but at the same time, that they are different.

And it is not that psychiatry is the means and mental health is the end. Cardiology services, for example, are not designated as "cardiology and cardiovascular health." This seems to be due rather to three reasons:

- The neuropsychiatric nature of the mental hygiene movement (precursor of mental health organizations and actions).
- Social matters are included within mental health problems that could hardly be considered a psychiatric pathology in a strict sense.
- The strong presence of professionals who do not come from a biomedical matrix in mental health.

Due to its proximity to public health, there is a tendency to think about promotional and preventive actions, which necessarily leads to going outside the health area. Taking the focus off patients to look towards the environment is called "the community."

However, that is not the case when generating plans, programs, allocating resources, calculating costs, etc. Mental health appears to be reduced to a series of disorders, termed "mental and behavioral." Mental health services, units, or departments usually delimit their range of action in a rather conventional way, based on a list of disorders that would be their specialty.

Rather a fuzzy boundary.

Not many years ago, epilepsies crossed the frontier of psychiatry towards neurology. And many voices argue that psychiatry should assume that it is nothing but a subspecialty of neurology, since, strictly speaking, there would be no mental disorders, as it would be brain dysfunctions, that is, neurological problems (Baker & Menken: 2001).

The coherence of this point of view must be recognized. While it may seem politically incorrect to deny mental health, in practice, most psychiatrists and not a few psychologists function as if this were the case. And it shouldn't be surprising; it is a logical derivation of modern medicine's path and the aspirations of leading figures in psychiatry history, such as Kahlbaum, Kraepelin, or Schneider.

Furthermore, it would be in continuity with Western medicine, in its Hippocratic-Galenic aspect. The discussion of whether the sick soul or only the body has that possibility, whether there are moral illnesses or are the effects of the corruption of the body, is very old.

This is also how, on the other frontier, some see the opening of a vast field of existential and social problems as the characteristic of psychiatry: "Psychiatrists are called upon to treat problems that the medical-industrial complex hardly responds to. Such problems – paradoxically – constitute the most 'novel' of the psychiatric in the health system" (Lolas: 2008, p. 97).

Beyond how psychiatry will resolve its internal differences, it is impossible to ignore the psychiatric imprint in any approach that is made today to mental health. As a branch of medicine, although it is rather implicitly, psychiatric practice equates health and normality, and normality to functionality.

For this reason, it is not surprising that for a long time, psychometrics has been the main source of links between psychologists and psychiatrists. Psychometric tests are parallel to laboratory tests in physical medicine, assuming that the mind is just another organ, invisible, but that it has its physiology. Therefore, its own rules.

Likewise, this allows us to understand the facility for psychiatrists to implement interventions to modify the environment: suggesting job changes, indicating vacations, promoting marital separations, etc. In a physiological conception of mental health, it is necessary to ensure that the organism is not over-demanded by the environment's demands.

Definitions that point to "internal balance" are, at heart, physiological. It should be remembered that physiology imposed the ideal of homeostasis, self-regulation, a proverb of health, and a guarantee of individual autonomy.

From this physiological approach also come all definitions of mental health that appeal to "functioning"; for example, when the WHO indicates that the positive perspective conceives mental health as the *optimal state of functioning*. Therefore, aspires to promote the qualities of the human being and facilitate their maximum potential development.

The key, or rather, what could make a difference within this perspective, is how mechanistic or without the subject a physiological conception of health can become. On the other hand, what would be the expected effects of the brain's balance or good functioning?

Sigmund Freud

At the same time, medicine was definitively becoming applied biology, and psychiatry left behind the moral treatment and any link with philosophy – succumbing to the pessimism of the Theory of Degeneration. A group of neurologists, faced with the mysteries of the so-called "neuroses," in particular hysteria, opted for psychogenesis and word treatments.

These are known works of Charcot, Janet, Breuer, and of course, Freud. And although the modern term psychotherapy is the creation of JH Bernheim – who intended the legitimate and conscious use of suggestion in the cure – it is only with psychoanalysis that psychotherapeutic practice begins to acquire its own and recognized status and logic.

Because?

What differentiates Freud from his predecessors is that he elaborates not only on an explanation and treatment for hysterical symptoms but general psychology, whose two fundamental pillars are the notion of the unconscious and the drive.

As the unconscious and the drive are part of the human condition, the gap between healthy and sick becomes blurred, and psychotherapy is no longer an exclusive offer for those who have a diagnosis.

On the other hand, while doctors discard the patient's word in search of objective signs, Freud insists on a clinic of listening, which puts the symptom and its interpretation at the center of the medical act.

This is because the symptoms would be speech, messages, which refer to unconscious desires for the subject. Desires that ultimately lead to an impossible search, while total satisfaction is forbidden for the human being.

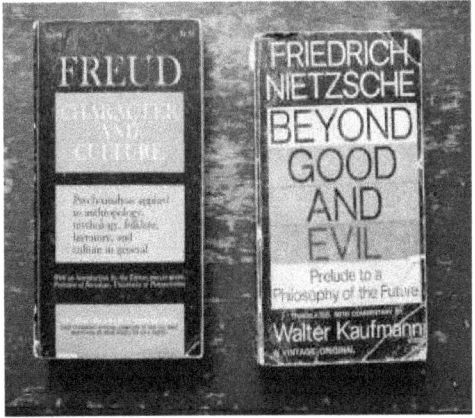

If in the beginning, mental health for Freud is in the possibility of making the unconscious conscious, which means subjecting the empire of reason to the fancies of passions ignored for the subject. Therefore, the paradoxical condition of the human being gives mental disorders an existential status.

Freud argues that the psychoanalytic cure offers are only better arrangements. Better in what way? In the possibility of enjoying and producing, loving, and working. This is how the mental health of an individual is known.

Freud is not alien to a physiological conception of health, insofar as he thinks of the mind as an "apparatus," with subsystems, instances, and functions. For the same reason, the difference between health and pathology would be somewhat quantitative.

But what psychoanalytic cure is about? In his late work, it is increasingly about knowing how to live, about having the fortitude and wisdom to take charge of being alive, a life that Freud was far from a paradise.

In other words, the therapeutic objective is closer to an ethical horizon, in the classic sense of the term, to a kind of knowing how to do with one's own life. So much so that those collaborators who later departed from Freud and created their psychotherapeutic currents, such as A. Adler, CG Jung,

Meanwhile, in the United States, the rise of the behaviorist movement made little relevance for psychologists and the psychological clinic, the very notion of mental health. The mind cannot be studied scientifically, nor does it seem necessary when explaining human behavior.

Behaviorism questions the concept of mental illness as an entity and maintains that what exists are maladaptive behaviors. That turn had an enormous impact on the psychological clinic, and therefore, on conceiving mental health.

Darwinism

It is known that American Academic Psychology, from functionalism onwards, including Psychoanalytic Psychology of the Ego and Cognitive Psychology, is strongly influenced by Darwin's ideas.

In this sense, you cannot talk about the individual's health without looking at the environment since health is measured in its ability to adapt to it. Normality aspiration loses weight, and health becomes rather synonymous with adaptation. Whether it is behaviors, the self, or cognitive schemas and processes, the north of all mental health treatment is to make the corresponding adjustments and corrections based on a better adaptation to the environment.

When you start to think in population terms, normality and adaptation are assimilated. Isn't it strange then that officially these psychotherapies are the best valued by government systems since they are close to medicine and education due to their corrective and normalizing nature? That's the question I ask the system.

Today, we can also see the continuity of these approaches with mental hygiene, which made its ideal of health the "social efficiency" (Lopera: 2012). It is quite different from what was proposed by the post-war WHO when it clarifies that the impulse to adapt to the environment is not in itself healthy and that, on the contrary, the healthy thing can be to change the environment.

It should be added that, in recent years, the same North American Academic Psychology, with the emergence of Positive Psychology, has shifted the horizon from adaptation to happiness, which otherwise seems to be the new object of public policies and the economy.

A correct life and a healthy mind produces a happy subject. Adaptation and happiness, then, could be the keys to defining mental health in official terms.

We could hardly deny the importance of a healthy organism of the capacity to respond to the environment's challenges in terms of adaptation. And happiness is in the Greco-Roman bases of Western culture, as what the human being can aspire to.

The question that arises, however, is because of the utilitarian connotations of this behavioral science. It evolves from a conception of the human being typical of said philosophy to a concern for the human being's usefulness as an instrument and drifts towards behavioral engineering. In the words of G. Canguilhem, the question that arises is: where do these psychologists want to go by doing what they do, and what role could a definition of mental health play in this?

Going back, it is necessary to recognize the impact of humanist psychology – the so-called 'Third Force' – in the United States itself and the world, which undoubtedly had direct consequences for psychotherapeutic work and the notion of mental health.

Although eclectic and quite vulnerable to fashions, humanistic psychology reintroduced the notion of human nature and trust in it. For this reason, each one is called to search within himself, in the real self or the organismic consciousness, the guidelines for a correct life. Mental health, then, is synonymous with congruence and spontaneity. According to what he is, a healthy person lives to the inner truth of his being, not to social roles or calculations of utility.

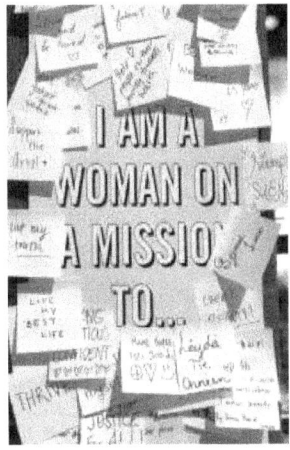

Humanists, in principle, depart from the adaptive and normalizing ideal of the psychotherapies of the 1950s. And rather, they seem to promote a return to classical ethics, to a dimension at least, which is not that of moderation, but rather that of doing what is following the ultimate nature as the way to be happy.

Living in harmony with your nature, that is, health. And with the arrival of transpersonal psychology, it is no longer just living in unity with our nature but living a life in union with the cosmic reality, destiny, or a kind of higher consciousness. The psyche is thus restored to its spiritual condition.

However, a somewhat different nuance arises when adding the notion of self-realization, so dear to humanist psychology, to the definition of mental health. The actualization of each one's potential as a key part of health is in different definitions of it. In contrast, mental health is inevitably impregnated with a developmental paradigm and the modern notion of progress.

Terms such as "grow as a person" or "personal development" are inseparable from the North American humanist current, which is usually interpreted as aspiring to more, having goals, going beyond the satisfaction of needs.

And it is that what we can understand as personal fulfillment is different in a worldview where everything has a place and tends towards something. What terms such as self-regulation, self-development, harmony, happiness, etc. imply. It will vary according to the cultural context in which they are promoted.

By way of synthesis and exaggerating things a bit, we can group psychotherapies, above the theories on which they are inspired, in two types of practices, and that point to two different types of mental health.

On one hand, some are inserted in a tradition that we can call ethical, or "spiritual," in the use that Michel Foucault makes of the expression in the course he dictates between 1981 and 1982 at the *College de France*, whose objective is close to something that we can call "practical wisdom."

On the other, psychotherapies that are better assimilated to medical or psychoeducation routines and whose objective would be to achieve the normalization and adaptation of the subjects to the social environment.

For the former, and continuing with Foucault, what is at stake is the subject's relationship with the truth and its transformation.

For the latter, what is at stake is the functionality of the individual. For the former, someone mentally healthy is someone who knows how to live their life.

For the latter, someone healthy is someone useful.

It is difficult and probably irrelevant for the former to objectify and measure mental health, even more so in a universal way.

For the latter, the concept of mental health can be conceived as a list of properties or characteristics according to a prototype that, if carefully examined, is beneficial for a given social, political, and economic system.

I am sorry if you are confused.

One issue that should cause some surprise within the health field is that many times, mental health is accompanied by expressions such as: "citizenship," "human rights," "democracy," or "social exclusion."

As has already been said, the boom in mental health begins with the post-war period and the need to generate political and social orientations that guarantee social peace. For this reason, it is not surprising that the First World Congress on Mental Health, which was held in London in 1948, had the motto: "Mental Health and Citizenship of the World."

We must not lose sight of the fact that mental health is part of the effort to create a new world order as we know it today. And the slogan of this new order is "biopsychosocial well-being" as a guarantor of peace.

The very concept of mental health has become political rather than technical or scientific. It is something that those critical movements that are born as an alternative to asylum psychiatry, either to disown the notion of mental health or to make use of it. It is about picking up without drama as a pivot to disregard the approach to mental problems and underline its link with social, economic, and cultural conditions.

Antipsychiatry, Social Medicine, and Community and Liberation Psychology in Latin America revitalize the concept of alienation, but no longer as the mental alienation of the 19th century, but as social alienation.

To define mental health, the individual-society relationship is again brought to the front. But the focus is no longer an individual maladaptive to the social environment, but the other way around. For example, a society that creates conditions for an alienated existence.

For this reason, on the horizon of these movements, there is the old idea of freedom. The mental is defined as a consequence of socio-economic structures, the material environment, and cultural life. Mental health is conceived "recursively related to the notion of global capital within a framework of rights and human development, as a problem of political and economic well-being." (Restrepo & Jaramillo: 2012, p. 206).

In the name of mental health, individualism and capitalism are criticized and dictatorships, discrimination, and inequality.

However, what is meant by mental health is rarely said. There is a little theoretical reflection on the concept. In practice, everything fits: interpellation to the State and state plans and programs, work with citizen associations, therapeutic communities, educational workshops, self-help groups, research-action, investigation statistics, etc.

As a theoretical infrastructure, there is considerable flexibility and eclecticism, resort to several concepts, such as self-confidence, self-esteem, empowerment, resilience, social capital, relational capital, psychosocial stress, quality of life, protective and risk factors, etc.

In general, there is more emphasis on action than on theory. Transversal is that it maintains a critical position towards biomedicine and a medical system of the assistance type, approaching public health due to the promotional and preventive emphasis. And due to the community discourse, it is increasingly aligned with official policies and epidemiology.

What is not clear among such an abundant repertoire of actions is what, specifically, it is that it is trying to promote. Perhaps without noticing it, it is implicitly ascribed to a physiological conception of mental health. Simultaneously, the pathogenic consequences of modern life are denounced, elements of the social and economic system that would be harmful to the individual, and general discomfort. Furthermore, it has a direct antecedent in Social Medicine and a long tradition in the social sciences.

There is no health without mental health.

Faced with the risk that mental health is reduced to a field of action of specific specialists who attend to a limited number of problems, the World Health Organization has endorsed the motto: "There is no health without mental health."

Although this can be criticized as a tautology or an unnecessary redundancy, we cannot ignore the impact of mind-body dualism in the health sciences and the divorce between the "bio" and the "psycho" and "social," which is not solved by writing the three terms together as if it were a magic formula.

The WHO, in the well-known 2001 World Health Report, says verbatim that mental health is understood as: subjective well-being, perception of one's efficacy, autonomy, competence, intergenerational dependence, and self-realization of intellectual and emotional capacities.

In the current Comprehensive Action Plan on Mental Health 2013-2020, the WHO defines mental health as "a state of well-being in which the individual realizes his capacities, overcomes the normal stress of life, works productively and fruitfully, and contributes something to their community."

A set of positively valued attributes are collected in a social environment like ours in both cases. However, it is worth dwelling on one particularity: these are, for the most part, questions that would hardly be required of an animal of another species.

Suppose, then, that mental health is what makes the difference between animal health and human health. It was only pertinent to speak of mental health for the human sphere. It would already be the first decision.

If so, mental health would be nothing more and nothing less than the human dimension of health. What would make the difference between a veterinarian and a doctor dedicated to the homo sapiens species? It inevitably leads us to philosophical anthropology. Since we would have to discuss what it is, that makes us human.

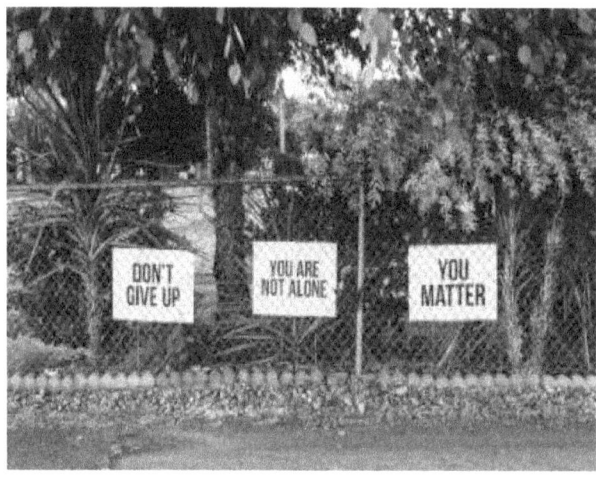

And it also brings us to psychology, since the historical separation between the field of the natural and the human, the world and the self, which incidentally enables the modern sciences to take off, leave medicine in charge of the bodily machinery.

Now, as there is not one psychology but several, we return to what we pointed out above, there is not only one way to approach mental health from psychology.

If mental health is a *complement* to true health, that of the body, there is a more or less easy way out of dealing with the *true illness* and the state of mind of the person who suffers it. That would be a possible translation for the slogan 'there is no health without mental health' and what is usually done in medical services.

However, it could go further and make that phrase an attempt to change the dominant conception of health. It would try to stop dissociating disease and sick, and for the same reason, to question an essentialist and reifying conception of diseases. And that no longer looks easy.

Everything that is constructed as 'evidence' today supposes an ontological conception of the disease. And in practice, the subject is no more relevant to the medical act than the setting for a play would be.

Under the heading of mental health, there is a huge amount of research, data, texts, projects, conferences, funds, etc., which is not consistent with the scant reflection on the notion of mental health itself. And it is even legitimate to think that it cannot be otherwise.

Many distrust the concept of mental health, as it always goes hand in hand with promoting a social ideal. And many times, with the attempt to measure and objectify something that is inevitably subjective, which could be inappropriate and even dangerous (Canguilhem: 2004). At the other extreme, there would be those for whom it makes no sense to talk about mental health since it can only make the body sick and heal.

Both positions have arguments in their favor. And yet there are numerous advocates or even activists for mental health. In the name of mental health, most of them seek to improve living conditions and promote democracy, equality, and human rights.

Health is an unquestionable ideal in our society and one of the few foundations that can be used to establish regulations and make changes in the economic, productive, and political fields. In this sense, the concept of mental health would have a strategic value as an argument in the political struggles of the so-called progressive sectors.

It could also have strategic value in attempts to curb biomedical colonization of the healthcare field. However, all this has its reverse. On the one hand, it is very easy to instrumentalize mental health to promote a type of subject with functional characteristics to a given political or economic system.

The great totalitarianism of the first half of the 20th century did. But we can also suspect that capitalist democracies use the concept of mental health to describe, in the end, a good worker and a good consumer. On the other hand, it is easy for daily life to be medicalized in the name of mental health. In other words, as a political instrument, it is a double-edged sword.

Chapter 4: The advent of empathy and emotional intelligence in our lives

Empathy, much more than putting yourself in someone else's shoes. We define empathy and explain why it is an essential quality for your life.

Empathy is one of the most important competencies that are included in emotional intelligence. The word comes from the Greek words that mean "inside him" and "what he feels." However, this psychological phenomenon's real meaning is even more important than the ability to put oneself in someone else's place.

What is empathy?

Empathy is the ability to understand the emotional life of another person, almost in all its complexity. This does not necessarily mean sharing the same opinions and arguments that justify the other person's state or reaction. It does not even mean agreeing with the interlocutor's way of interpreting emotionally charged situations.

Empathy refers, among other things, to active listening, understanding, and emotional support. Also, empathy implies having enough capacity to differentiate between others' affective states and the ability to take perspective, both cognitive and affective, to the person who expresses his emotional state to us.

It's components

Perhaps you have not felt heard on some occasions due to a lack of feedback, support, or understanding. On many other occasions, you may feel that you have not been able to adequately and empathically attend to the emotional state of the other person and ask yourself:

What do I need, or should I do to be more empathetic?

Fundamentally, the components of empathy are the following:

1. Know how to listen

Pay attention to what the other person explains or argues, pay attention to non-verbal manifestations, as it would be in the case of gestures that correspond to the state of mind that is verbalized and do not interrupt the verbal discourse.

Besides, reflect on what the other person is communicating to you and express active follow-up signals as feedback: look at the face, nod your head, or reflect facial expressions congruent with what the other person is explaining to you.

On the other hand, it is necessary to show interest by asking details about the conversation's content.

2. Interpret non-verbal cues

It includes the transmitted messages of a paralinguistic nature, such as intonation, response time, volume.

3. Show understanding

We can show a harmonious understanding of what they explain to us through phrases such as: "I understand that you acted like this. "I understand how you feel." "The truth is that you must have had a great time" ...

The emotions of the person who expresses them should not be invalidated, rejected, or judged, as this is a fundamental premise to show empathic sensitivity.

4. Give emotional help if needed

It is important always to ask our interlocutor if you need any kind of help. However, on many occasions, simply by actively listening to the other, we allow them to "air" and manage their emotional state. In this way, he is relieved to have a reliable listener to whom to convey his emotions.

When the person who listens empathically has lived an emotional situation similar to the one expressed, the communication process is more fluid since there is a greater emotional harmony.

Why practice emotional intelligence?

- As an emotional intelligence ability, empathy is important because it makes it possible to experience various advantages.
- It enables you to appreciate social relationships by interacting more with peers, coworkers, or family groups.
- It makes you feel better.
- Facilitates settlement of disputes.
- It predisposes others to support and share.
- Increases charisma and appeal.
- Let's be politer.

Developing expertise in teamwork, negotiation, and cooperation, as well as becoming better regarded by others.

How can empathy be cultivated?

Empathy practice allows us to widen our viewpoints and enrich our world with new thoughts, points of view, and possibilities.

As we have already shown, it is a vital social ability that helps us listen better, comprehend, and ask better questions, three essential aspects of effective communication. Furthermore, it is one of the pillars of establishing powerful and enriching relationships.

You can incorporate three simple, practical exercises into your routine to improve your empathy.

1. Ask and show interest

Start any meeting or conversation with open and personalized questions: How are you? How about at work? How is the project you started doing? How were your vacations?

Showing closeness and interest in the other person leave room for them to open up and simply receive.

2. Read theater scripts

Read theater scripts and focus on one character. Search the text for what is beyond words; The personal history, previous experiences, the fears it hides, its desires and illusions, the emotions on the surface.

3. Choose a person

Choose a person at random and try to find out what moves them through their non-verbal communication (emotion and thought). A good time to carry out this exercise is in public transport, in a cafeteria. These places are rich in scenes as they can be used to put empathy into practice.

Are you empathetic? Ten typical traits of empathic people

Are you an empathetic person? Know that you also have some difficulties in dealing with it.

The characteristic feature of empathic people is that they know how to put themselves in others' shoes and understand their emotions and physical symptoms. They are extraordinarily sensitive people.

Their vision of the world is very intuitive. They relate to others prioritizing their emotions and sensations over calculation and coldness. They usually find it difficult to describe and put into words everything they feel.

Empathy: a quality to develop

Being an empathetic person is something positive for life. But it also has quite a few less desirable points. People with this trait may also be more vulnerable to the emotional impact of things around them.

For example, they may be more prone to anxiety attacks, depression, chronic fatigue, and other symptoms and disorders related to emotional instability.

However, empathy is a virtue that can help us a lot throughout life, especially if we learn to manage it effectively. The first step is to know if you are an empathic person.

The ten traits of empathy

This section describes the ten characteristic features (habits, attitudes, and behaviors) of people who have highly developed empathy.

1. They are more sensitive than other people

Empathic individuals are detached, open to new experiences, kind, and good "listeners." They are attentive people and know how to transmit these good feelings when communicating with others.

They are always ready to help and offer a shoulder to cry on. But they can also be hurt and offended with amazing ease. They are very sensitive people, to the point of being truly susceptible in some cases.

2. Empaths "absorb" the emotions of others

People with high empathy are influenced by other people's emotions and humor, for better or worse.

They can feel what others feel more vividly than ordinary people, which can sometimes be difficult to overcome. If they are around someone anxious or stressed, it is hard for them not to have their minds emulate those attitudes. Luckily, they are also infected with positive emotions.

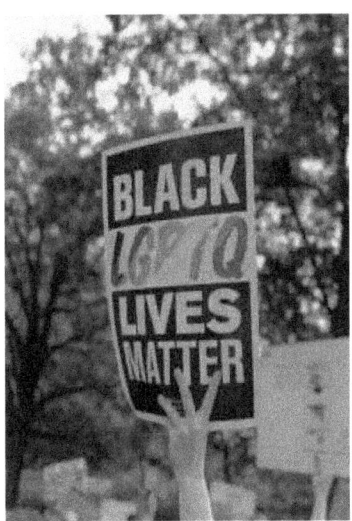

3. They are usually introverted

We can refer to the difference between introverts and extroverts. In the case of empathic people, it is often the case that they tend to be quite introverted. They don't enjoy large parties too much, preferring small groups or going out for coffee with a single friend.

Even among empathic subjects who are more open to going to parties and places with many people, they tend to be careful and prefer to moderate the amount of time they spend in these types of environments.

4. They are more intuitive than average

Empaths perceive the world through their intuition. They like to develop their intuition and listen to their hunches regularly. This allows them to surround themselves with positive people and get away from those who may upset their emotional balance.

5. They like to spend time alone

They are very sensitive people and tend to be affected if they are listening and helping others for a long time. For this reason, they periodically need to be alone to return to their emotional balance.

6. They can overprotect themselves in romantic relationships

Living with a partner can be complicated for an empathic person, and they can even develop Philophobia or similar manifestations. They avoid falling in love with someone, so they don't have to suffer later if things don't go quite right.

They may be afraid of being emotionally swallowed up by their partner. They need to redefine their concept of love relationship to have positive and happy relationships.

7. They are easy prey for emotional vampires

Have you heard of emotional vampires? They are those people who have a bad habit of unloading all their negativity on other people, from whom they "suck" their energy to continue in their spiral of fatalism, anger, and resentment.

Empathic people can especially suffer the effects of having an emotional vampire around, as they are especially vulnerable to all the bad feelings that these individuals convey.

8. They feel very comfortable in contact with nature

The obligations and stress of daily routines affect us all, but especially empathetic men and women. They tend to disconnect and recharge their batteries when surrounded by nature: climbing mountains, enjoying a sunny beach or simply strolling through a green meadow.

9. They have the sensations on the surface

Empathic people are more sensitive in general. They can feel very bad in noisy surroundings or when they notice that there is a lot of tension in the environment.

10. They are good people, even to the detriment of their well-being

Empathic individuals are good people - they have big hearts and sincerely care about others. They feel bad when they see someone suffering on the street, and they cannot help but attend to them to try to mitigate their pain.

Although it is an undeniable virtue, the truth is that empathic people can go too far and become obsessed with dealing with the problems of others and feel frustrated or confused if they cannot solve their problems.

Manage empathy

As we have seen, empathic people have a series of virtues associated with other problems for their emotional well-being.

Some techniques can help these people to manage their personalities and not be greatly damaged by their sensitivity. Controlling time and schedule, setting boundaries with people who need help, and habits like meditation and mindfulness can restore psychological well-being.

In this busy world we live in, in which we are constantly connected to new technologies, the mind jumps from one place to another continuously, scattering our thoughts and emotions, making us feel stressed, nervous, and even anxious.

The way of life in Western societies puts us on *automatic pilot*, which means that days go by without noticing what is happening inside or around us. We are pulling, walking through life, without stopping for a single moment to observe ourselves internally, without stopping to think about our needs. Always ruminating, clinging to expectations rather than reality.

Living on autopilot, a bad option

Living on autopilot, living by inertia, and being carried away by routine can be very comfortable in the short term. It's easier for the days to go by, and don't face the fear of talking to your partner about how you feel. Or is it less complicated to get carried away from day to day than to admit that you are sad, right? The planets will align to solve your problems.

But living far from the present, that is, with the armor on and without feeling anything, can be negative in the long run, because when something happens, that shakes us (for example, we are fired from work or our partner leaves us), then we have to step on with feet on the ground. Also, living up to expectations can make us wildly unhappy.

Mindfulness: more than techniques, a philosophy of life

More than a set of techniques to be in the present moment, mindfulness practice is a philosophy of life, an attitude that must be adopted to reconnect with oneself. It is a coping style that boosts personal strengths, helps self-regulate behavior, get to know each other better, and creates an environment conducive to well-being.

In other words, mindfulness is a conscious and intentional way of tuning in to what is happening within us and around us and allows us to unmask automatisms and promote integral development.

A few minutes a day is not so much...

For some people, those who live eternally stressed, finding 5 minutes a day to connect with yourself can be difficult. But investing 10, 15, or 20 minutes a day for your well-being is not so much.

As already mentioned, the important thing in this discipline's practice, regardless of the techniques used, is to adopt the Mindfulness attitude, which promotes attention in the present moment, without judging, and with compassion towards oneself and towards oneself and others.

5 Mindfulness exercises for greater well-being

Before going to the list of exercises, it is important to note that practicing mindfulness, being an attitude towards life, is not limited simply to performing these exercises but is a way of dealing with the events that occur in daily life. Still, adopting a healthy habit like this is beneficial for many reasons.

With that said, here is a list of practical Mindfulness exercises:

1. Mindfulness in a single minute

This exercise is ideal if you are starting to practice mindfulness as you progress in learning mindfulness. It is ideal for increasing practice until you reach about 15 or 20 minutes a day. Also, because it only takes one minute, this exercise can be practiced anywhere and at any time in your daily life.

2. Landing breath here and now

This exercise is ideal for turning off the autopilot. By practicing it, your attention is focused on the present moment and stops the constant flow of thoughts, memories, images, or ideas. It is ideal for discharging the accumulated tension in a very simple way.

To do this, you need to focus your attention on your breath. A gentle, deep, and constant inspiration should be taken through the nose. When filling ourselves with air, immediately release the air through the mouth with intensity but without forcing the throat. Noticing a distraction (which is normal), we observe what caught our attention, and we return to the breath.

3. Mindfulness breakfast

It is common to get up in the morning on autopilot. You get out of bed, shower, get dressed, eat breakfast, brush your teeth, and another day at work. Yes, another day!

You can break this negative habit by doing mindfulness in the morning. So you will face the day differently. For this, you must sit in a quiet place and turn off the television so that you are silent. You must also have the mobile away. It's about not having distractions. When you get ready to have breakfast, try to focus your attention on the flavors, smells, the touch of food, or drink... feel them! In this way, you will be with your attention in the present moment, and you will see the difference.

4. Attention to the sounds of the moment

This exercise consists of consciously observing the sounds that occur in our environment. Therefore, it is about staying listening, hearing them as they sound without identifying them, judging them as pleasant or unpleasant, or thinking about them. Without any effort, sounds are observed, and other external perceptions are put aside. When noticing a distraction, we observe what captured our attention, and we return to listening to the sounds, relying exclusively on the breath of that moment.

When listening to sounds that enter our ears, thoughts, and feelings related to what we hear arise. This exercise tries to know silence and sound in a not conceptual way (without thinking) but experientially (feeling them).

5. Body scanner

With this exercise, we try to get in touch with our body's experience as it is, without judging, without rejecting the unpleasant sensations or sticking to the pleasant ones. This exercise is also called a body sweep or body scan.

It is necessary to sit in a comfortable position, with an upright back, although it is also possible to adopt the lying position. Then close your eyes, pay attention to your breathing, and walk through your body. This type of meditation is advisable to be guided.

8 Mindfulness activities to improve emotional health

A selection of practical mindfulness exercises for both children and adults.

Mindfulness, or mindfulness, is one of the most useful tools to achieve emotional balance and improve people's concentration and well-being.

Its effectiveness has been scientifically proven, and there is increasing evidence that its use helps regulate emotions, reduce stress and anxiety, help you sleep better, and promote creativity. Mindfulness is also enriching for those healthy people without psychological imbalances, who simply want to live their life more fully.

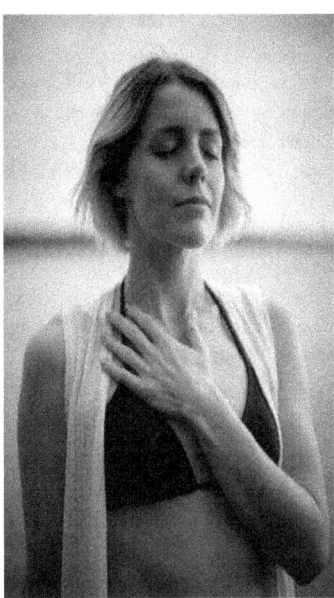

This ancient practice allows you to be in the present moment. It is a coping style that fosters personal strengths and helps to be more aware of the immediate experience with a non-judgmental, open, and accepting attitude. Mindfulness helps self-regulate behavior and promotes self-awareness, as well as creating an ideal environment for well-being.

Mindfulness activities for greater emotional balance

But more than a set of techniques to be in the present moment, mindfulness is a philosophy of life. This attitude must be adopted to reconnect with oneself and be more aware of the reality surrounding us. It requires practice and will, so it is necessary to carry out a series of activities to improve the ability to be in the here and now with a non-judgmental and compassionate mindset.

There are many exercises for this purpose. Below you can find a series of mindfulness activities for children and adults.

Children can also get started in mindfulness practice. In this way, they develop this habit that will help them know each other better and relate better to the environment to be happier in the future.

1. Bee breathing

The Bee Breath, or Bhramari Pranayama, is a simple but very effective exercise to focus attention on the breath and to free the mind from agitation, frustration, anxiety, and get rid of anger. Since its practice is not very complex, it can be done anywhere and even at an early age. It consists of covering the ears, closing the eyes, and exhaling the air. It is necessary to pronounce the letter "m" until the breath is finished.

Without a doubt, it is an easy exercise to practice, although it is necessary to learn diaphragmatic breathing to be able to exhale for longer. The exercise can be done as many times as you want, but it is advisable to start with few repetitions and gradually increase them. The sound that results from this action is similar to the buzzing of a bee. That is why this activity is called "Bee Breathing."

2. The art of playing

To perform this exercise, it is necessary to place the children in pairs. One of them is given an object (a pen, a toy, a stone, a ball, etc.) and is asked to close his eyes. The child who has the object describes it to his partner.

After a minute or two, the same process is carried out, but this time, the other partner is in charge of describing the object. Despite this activity's simplicity, it is ideal for teaching the little ones that they can isolate their senses and, if they wish, they can focus their attention to live different experiences.

3. Attention to the hood

This exercise has two parts. The first one consists of ringing a bell and asking the children to listen to the vibration of the sound of it. Little ones should listen carefully and raise their hands when they no longer hear the sound vibration. Afterward, they should be silent for a minute and pay attention to the other sounds heard after the ringing of the bell has stopped.

When the sound ends, the children should be encouraged to share their experiences and say what they heard during this period. This activity works attention and mindfulness and helps to connect with the here and now.

4. Become a frog

Children can learn to practice mindfulness by turning into a frog for a few minutes. Frogs are a clear example of what mindfulness is. Just like when people meditate, frogs remain motionless for a long time. They are rarely agitated but stand still, watching and breathing calmly, and their belly moves sharply with each inhales and exhale. By adopting this amphibian role, children learn to stay still, breathe in a controlled manner, and observe what is happening around them without flinching.

...and for adults

Adults can practice mindfulness in their everyday lives practically anywhere. Any time is a good time to focus on the present moment, adopt a non-judgmental mindset, and treat yourself with compassion.

5. Exercise of the five senses

This exercise is simple and can be applied quickly in almost any situation. All it takes is being aware of our senses and experiencing each of them separately. To perform this activity, you just have to follow this order:

- Look at **five things you can see**. Look around you and pick something you wouldn't normally notice, like a shadow or a small crack in the ground.
- Observe **four things you can feel**. Become aware of four things that you are feeling in the present moment, such as the texture of the pants, the feeling of the breeze on your skin, or the smooth surface of the table where you are resting your hands.
- Look at **three things you can hear** and focus on the sounds around you. For example, a bird, the refrigerator's noise, or the sound of traffic on a nearby highway.
- Notice **two things you can smell**. Pay attention to smells that you are generally unaware of and see if they are pleasant or unpleasant. The smell of nearby pine trees, of the beach if you live on the coast, or of a fast-food restaurant near your house.
- Observe **the taste of your mouth**. Focus on the taste of the present moment. You can sip a drink that you have on hand, chew gum, eat something, and even taste the taste of your mouth without ingesting anything.

This is an easy exercise to practice that can quickly take you to the here and now. How long you spend with each sense is up to you, but each object of attention should last a minute or two. The idea **is not to do meditation but to return to the present with an improved state of consciousness**.

6. Active listening: observe non-verbal language

This activity is ideal for developing active listening skills, a form of communication that requires an effort on the part of our cognitive and empathic capacities. The receiver is not a mere receiver of the words of the sender. Many times, we think we are listening when we are hearing.

Active listening is not listening to the other person but being focused on the message that the other individual is trying to communicate. It is being in the here and now with full awareness. We focus not only on the speaker's words but also on what they are trying to convey through non-verbal language.

To perform this exercise, it is necessary to get in pairs. One member has two minutes to explain a pleasant experience in their life or an opinion on a recent event, while the other actively listens. What do your eyes, your posture, or your gestures say? Do you seem proud when you tell? Does it convey passion? The receiver has two minutes to observe the non-verbal communication of his partner carefully. After finishing the exercise, both share their experience as active listeners.

7. Mindfulness eating

With the rhythm of life, we have today, it is usual that we do not stop for a moment to connect with ourselves, not even when we have a few minutes to eat, because either we turn on the television or we are thinking about what we have to do this afternoon. Well, it is possible to practice mindfulness while we eat or have breakfast. To do the mindful eating exercise, you simply have to pay full attention to what you will eat.

You can start by focusing on what you are holding. Observe the feeling of what you have in your hands (for example, a toast or a fork). Once you know the texture, weight, color, etc., focus your attention on the smell. Finally, put the food in your mouth, but do it slowly and with full awareness. Notice the taste or texture as it melts in your mouth. This activity can help you discover new experiences with foods that you frequently eat.

8. Attention to the center of the image

To carry out this activity, it is necessary to view the audiovisual content shown below:

This exercise's objective is simple: to focus attention on the point that is visualized in the center of the image despite the changing color pattern around it, which can become distracting or provoke unwanted thoughts. It is an ideal exercise to start in the practice of mindfulness and become aware of the thoughts that come to mind and are sometimes not aware.

This exercise aims not to get lost in these thoughts, which can be very pronounced in people prone to anxiety. This experience is similar to the phenomenon of silent fixation that results from staring at a candle flame.

Work and organizational psychology: a profession with a future

Psychologists in companies, their functions, and their importance for the health of corporations.

Many students start their degree in psychology, thinking about dedicating themselves to clinical psychology. Still, as the profession progresses, they find that dedicating themselves to that field of psychology is increasingly difficult. One of the areas with the greatest career prospects is the psychology of work and organization, of which many psychologists become part of a company's human resources department.

However, human resources and organizational psychology are not quite the same, and becoming a specialist in human resources is not a prerequisite for becoming a psychologist. On the other hand, in addition to the human resources department, an organizational psychologist may perform his duties at the management level or in the field of commercial research and marketing and even development.

In today's section, we will review the organizational psychologist functions, and we will delve into the differences between it and the human resources professional.

The work or organization *psychologist*, also known as *an industrial psychologist* or business *psychologist*, is a professional who applies psychology principles in the organizational and works environment.

To do this, he has studied mental processes and human behavior (both individual and group) and puts into practice his training for problem-solving in the workplace. Its general role encompasses the study, diagnosis, coordination, intervention, and human behavior management within organizations.

You can work as part of the company as an employee within its organizational chart (for example, in the selection and training department). However, sometimes, you can work as part of an external company outside the organization. Performing functions of evaluating the performance, work environment, and health of workers or offering coaching services for employees or managers, among other functions. Some organizational psychologists choose to develop their professional careers as scientists or teachers.

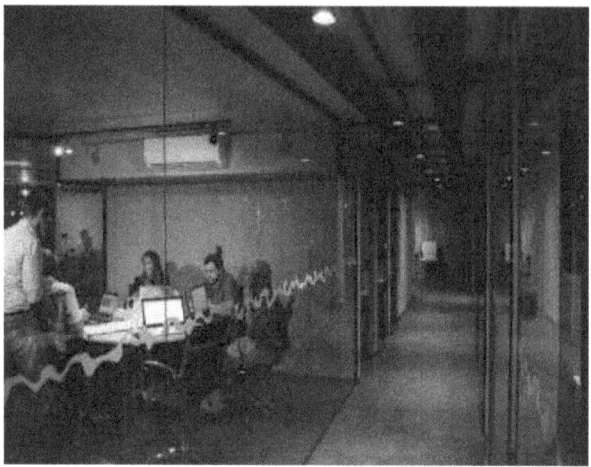

On the other hand, this concept is closely related to work psychology, although some nuances differentiate them. As its name suggests, organizational psychology focuses on the interactions between individuals, those who make up a team, a company, a department, etc. On the other hand, work psychology focuses on work dynamics, that is, the application of strategies and behavior patterns to start from a series of available resources to obtain a specific and objectively observable result: a product, a plan, a service, etc.

Functions of the work or organizational psychologist

The organizational or work psychologist has an important role in three main areas:

- **Human Resources** (education, training, etc.)
- **Marketing** and Social and Commercial Research.
- **Occupational Health and Safety** (Occupational Health Psychology)

But what are the functions it performs? Some of the functions of this professional are the following:

- **Plans, organizes or directs various functions within the organization**, such as recruiting, evaluating, compensating, retaining, and developing people.
- **Observe, describe, analyze, diagnose, and resolve conflicts** in human interactions. In this way, it ensures a good work environment and develops the organizational culture.
- **Analyze and modify the physical, social, and psychological elements** that affect job performance and impact employees' efficiency.
- **Apply questionnaires and interviews for the correct diagnosis of the climate**, productivity, and occupational health, and carry out preventive actions to correct possible imbalances.

- **When necessary**, advise the scorecard regarding collective bargaining, possible business strategies, improvement of corporate image, etc.
- **Analyze and put into practice different psychological techniques** to increase productivity, improve the organizational climate, avoid fatigue, and anticipate accidents or occupational health problems, such as **burnout**.
- **He contributes his knowledge as an expert in leadership styles**, interpersonal relationships, emotional control, negotiation techniques, decision-making, or correct planning.
- **It uses tools for talent detection and organizational development improvement** and conducts studies on consumer needs.
- **Recommend and implement actions to incentivize, compensate, and remunerate** staff and ensure their well-being, safety, and occupational health.
- **He is in charge of the training area and designs training programs** for staff development and career and promotion plans.
- **Directs and executes the personnel selection processes**. To do this, you can use different psychological tests and questionnaires to detect the candidates' competencies.
- **Analyze the needs of the staff**, the job, and the organization.

Differences between the occupational psychologist and the human resources professional

It is common to refer to the organizational psychologist as the human resources professional when they are different. The organizational psychologist is a psychologist who has specialized in the field of organizations and work, while the human resources professional may not have training as a psychologist.

The subjects taught in this career include occupational psychology subjects and other subjects, such as labor and trade union law or taxation of individuals.

This occurs because in the human resources department of a company, personnel selection or training functions are carried out, and collective negotiations or tasks such as payroll management can be carried out. The organizational psychologist's profile fits into some areas of this human resources department, but not all.

Organizational psychologist training

Suppose you are a psychologist and want to dedicate yourself to organizational psychology. In that case, you should know that an organizational psychologist, unlike the human resources professional, has completed a Degree in Psychology. Some psychologists finish their degree and then start working as recruiters or recruitment technicians. After learning about the world of human resources, they are trained to cover other HR areas, such as personnel administration or labor law.

Others, on the other hand, after finishing the Degree in Psychology, decide to do a master's degree. If that is your intention, you must choose between taking a master's in human resources management or a Master's in Organizational and Work Psychology.

While the first one trains you on issues such as budget, personnel payments, and expenses, labor legislation, contracts, labor rights, worker safety systems (avoid accidents) selection, and training, the second allows you to study the behavior of the individual within an organization and everything related to motivation, leadership, stress (and other work-related illnesses), work climate and culture or the influence of psychological variables on performance.

The most common psychological problems in top executives

These are the most common psychopathologies among senior executives and managers. People under high pressure are more likely to develop certain psychological disorders. This is the case of senior executives, managers, and other highly responsible positions.

Below we will compile the most common diagnoses that usually occur in this type of person due to their jobs and lifestyle characteristics.

What are the most common psychopathologies among senior executives?

Executives, managers, and other profiles of the highest business level are subjected to daily routines that facilitate the appearance of a series of pathologies. Let's see what the most common psychological problems in senior executives and related positions are.

1. Anxiety

It is not surprising that the first psychological pathology that we encounter when talking about people who live by and their work is anxiety. These individuals will tend to live in a constant state of alert, continually anticipating possible situations related to their work environment and the decisions they have to make to always achieve the best results.

This over-activation, logically, is not something that the body or mind can endure for a sustained time without a series of consequences, some physical and others psychological. The most common psychological symptoms of anxiety are a constant feeling of guilt, worry, and overwhelm. Sometimes you can fear the loss of control and even think that you may die.

Among the most common psychological problems in senior executives, anxiety causes these people to be restless, irritable, have trouble concentrating, and feel like they forget some things. They can also experience blockages at the motor level, which feeds back anxiety, establishing a vicious circle.

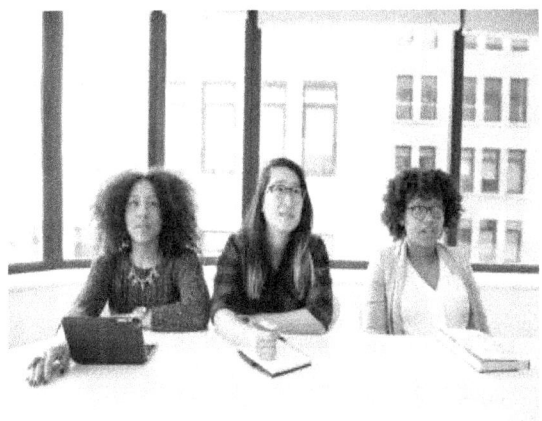

2. Depression

Depression is, along with anxiety, one of the most frequent mental disorders. Hence, it is logical to think that it is another of the most common psychological problems in senior executives. It is not uncommon for the two to appear together since the Anxious-depressive symptomatology is one of the pictures that psychologists often find in their consultations.

Depression is characterized by **a mood of general sadness, feelings of guilt, and unhappiness**, sometimes due to a traumatic event and other times without a clear cause, but which can perfectly fit with an exhausting lifestyle that ends up exhausting the mental defenses of the individual. The case of senior managers would be a profile in which this disease could emerge if the necessary precautions are not taken to avoid it.

3. Obsessive-compulsive disorder

Another of the most common psychological problems in senior executives would be OCD or obsessive-compulsive disorder, which would be related to anxiety disorders but with very specific characteristics. Hence the DSM-5 diagnostic manual gives it a category Independent. In this case, **people develop a series of irrational obsessions that they try to appease through compulsive behaviors**.

These obsessions or circular thoughts saturate these individuals' minds, preventing them from focusing on other issues normally, so they develop rituals or compulsions to try to leave those thoughts behind and be able to focus on the issues that concern them. For a person like a manager who needs his mental capacity to the maximum, intrusive thoughts represent a big problem.

OCD is not a disease that affects as much population as anxiety itself. Still, it is common for those people who have a greater propensity to suffer it to see it even more facilitated by a high level of stress maintained over time, which is precisely the lifestyle that a manager usually leads. Hence this is one of the most common psychological problems in senior executives.

4. Narcissistic personality disorder

The fourth psychological alteration that we would find would be a narcissistic personality disorder. In this case, we are talking about a psychological alteration that affects the person's personality that **makes him perceive himself with importance beyond what it corresponds to**. The individual who suffers from this disorder usually believes himself to be the center of the world, with qualities few or no one else possesses.

Not only that, but you need others to make you see how special you are so that compliments will be almost a requirement. This feeling also **causes him to consider that his rights are greater than those of others**, and therefore he will expect better treatment than anyone else, simply because he is who he is.

You will have little or no empathy and expect your subordinates to be 100 percent involved in company tasks, regardless of their personal lives, health, or other issues. Indeed, it is a profile that could fit some senior managers in some companies, so narcissistic personality disorder could not be absent as one of the most common psychological problems in senior executives.

What elements of the professional context generate these alterations?

After addressing the most common psychological problems in senior executives, we must know the bases that make these people have a greater tendency to suffer certain pathologies than the rest of the population. We are talking about **the profile of a person who usually works many more hours a day than would make up a typical workday**, which is generally 8 hours.

On the other hand, these individuals may spend 10, 12, or even 14 hours in the office. It is also common for them to move between different venues, sometimes internationally, which implies traveling by plane, sometimes even changing time zones, with the consequent jet lag. Timing is everything, and they generally rush from one place to another to get to all the meetings on time and have several on the same day.

Besides, **this implies a very poor sleep**, supplemented with large doses of coffee, which only acts as a patch, since nothing works the same as restful sleep. Not only is it the lack of sleep, but it is also that this situation is usually accompanied by fairly improvable nutrition, because sometimes because not a single minute of work is wasted, the intake is done very quickly or sometimes it does not even take place, which is even worse.

As if that were not enough, the issues dealt with at the work level on a day-to-day basis are highly sensitive, involving making decisions of enormous significance, which can mean a rise or fall in the company's stock market, million-dollar profits or losses, and achieve closing deals essential with other companies or even have in their hands the possibility of winning or losing projects that involve many jobs.

Handling all of these issues constantly is something that not all minds are ready to do. Even the strongest can suffer a series of consequences, which are some of the most common psychological problems in top executives and which we have previously seen in detail.

The last factor would be that of free time. **The disconnection from work, so important to clear the mind after a tiring day at work**, many executives do not have. Endless days at the office are followed by moments at home in which this person does not disconnect. You use your phone or computer to answer calls or emails, review documents, or try to move forward on different projects.

The same thing happens during the holidays. These individuals never really disconnect from work because they think that their tasks are essential for the company, and therefore they do not usually take days off. If they do, the same thing happens when they get home: they are watching their laptop or their smartphone, so they simply move their workstation to another location.

This factor also affects their personal and family lives. Sometimes they have problems getting involved as much as they would like and thus enjoy more time and with better quality, for example with their children, their partners, their friends, etc. This could enhance the discomfort that the person already feels with the situation, as it would affect him to involving third parties.

In summary, I am talking about people with responsibilities of the highest level, who travel constantly, sleep little, do not have healthy eating habits, hardly know how to disconnect, with hardly any vacations or free time with their own family. It seems like an extraordinary breeding ground to generate a whole series of pathologies that we have seen, representing the most common psychological problems in top executives.

Chapter 5: Emotional intelligence in design and marketing

Cartesian dualism has marked our way of understanding emotion as an independent aspect of mental processes. The latest studies in the neurological field allow us to understand the fundamental role of emotions in information processing. This section reviews the latest trends in marketing, advertising, and design that reflect this new way of understanding the brain.

The new currents of *marketing* and communication, such as *one-to-one marketing* or relationship *marketing*, have raised trust as a theoretical basis to foster friendly relationships with consumers.

This new way of understanding *marketing* is based on four trends that have been decisive in the genesis and conception of unconventional communication: interactive communication, relationship, loyalty, and permission.

The goal is to achieve customer loyalty always to buy the same brand because they are convinced of their superiority over the competition. This ideal situation is increasingly difficult to achieve since the products are more like each other, and the differences are hardly noticeable:

The fading of the product identity of the product due to the constant technological change intervention that continuously modifies it already the loss of objective differences (in their components, their applications, etc.) between the goods of different manufacturers.

The consumer takes the product's quality for granted and wants to trust a brand that offers guarantees. For this reason, companies consider it more profitable to keep current customers, who already know the product, than to convince potential customers through large advertising budgets.

In this sense, the brand is constituted as a set of intangibles that give meaning to the product's material value.

The brand's main role is to create and spread a universe of significance around a social object (be it a product, good, or service). This brand universe confers personality and character to the product, which allows us to differentiate it.

Thus, decide more in line with our scale of values. Even certain brands have created such a solid universe that they arouse both sympathies and antipathies in society, thus equating themselves with political parties or religious institutions. For this reason, more and more brands are made up of subjective attributes, also called emotional:

Normally these values are defined in opposition to the materials or functional and receive different names according to the authors. We can designate them as "implicit, subjective and immaterial values" or as "sensorial-emotional experience" and simply as "emotion."

From this point of view, emotional values are built independently of the functional value of the product. This responds to a classic conception of the relationship between reason and emotion, as opposing values can never be combined, as autonomous functions of the brain.

However, scientific advances in recent decades, especially in the neurological field, have shown that emotional processes take place in the brain, in the same way as rational processes, interacting with each other,

For this reason, an analysis of emotion is essential as a transversal concept of the brand, from the design of the product to its communication. To do this, we must know the origin of the importance of emotional values in the communicational field and its implication with other disciplines such as neuroscience and industrial engineering.

Humanization of communication

The beginning of applying the so-called emotional values in the advertising campaigns of the big brands is the result of a deeper process of change that has changed the way of conceiving the consumer-company relationship. This treatment tries to imitate certain aspects of personal relationships based on trust and mutual respect. Both concepts are key in new disciplines, such as customer relationship management and permission marketing.

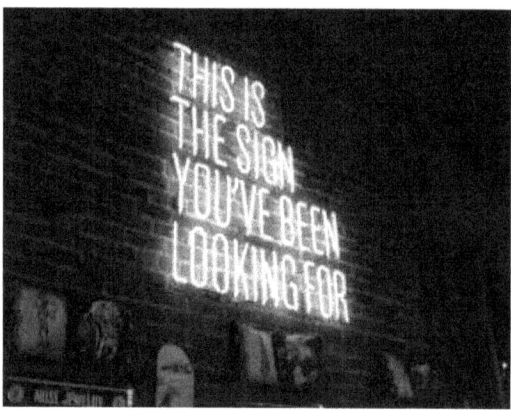

The humanization of communication is a real trend that is present in the main current theoretical currents. This coincides with the explosion of new technologies that offer users the necessary power to exercise their right to reply. Tools such as the Internet and the mobile phone have fostered interpersonal relationships by overcoming distance and space barriers.

The maximum expression of this trend is viral *marketing*. This communication strategy aims to professionalize traditional word of mouth by using interpersonal communication tools, especially email and mobile phones.

The main evidence of this fact is the proliferation of *marketing* campaigns viral and the birth of advertising agencies specialized in communication. However, this professionalization has led to a certain deviation naturally and spontaneously in which messages are spread. In this way, some brands offer material rewards to those who speak well of their products; others go further: they carry out orchestrated campaigns. They hire people who walk around with the product as regular consumers.

This manipulation could affect the confidence of the issuing source to the extent that there is an interest in launching the message.

Although *viral marketing* is not the subject of this section, it serves as an example to show how companies seek new ways to achieve a lasting relationship based on trust. This shows the difficulty that some brands find to connect with their consumers.

One of the traditional mistakes made by companies in their market analysis is the consideration of their target audience simply as a consumer of the brand, forgetting that they are people and customers.

In short, what has marked the beginning of a new stage in current communication is the passage from the importance of the product to the importance of the person, from the rational to the emotional. Although

Levitt already stated in the 60s in his famous section "*Marketing* myopia," where he highlighted the error of many companies when defining the objectives of the company, focusing more on the characteristics of products than on the needs they satisfy.

This humanization of communication strategies is a reality that today we can verify simply by contemplating any advertising *spot*, where more and more we find brands that seek identification with a series of global values, such as freedom in the campaigns of the telecommunications company Amena or the emotion in those of Movistar.

The consumer: the brand evangelizer

In contrast to this trend towards the humanization of communication, some authors maintain a new type of customer that is more demanding and concerned about the responsibility of their commercial actions.

This would mean thinking that people act rationally and thoughtfully when deciding to buy any product or service, considering its characteristics. At the same time, this contrasts with the lack of time and lack of interest, which forces decisions to be made quickly and without thought.

The excess of information and the lack of time to convert that information into true knowledge provoke in people a state of anxiety called information anxiety.

Is the customer as rational as we think? Do you make decisions after considering all aspects of the products or services you purchase? In general, we can say that the degree of involvement in the purchase decision process will depend on the type of product, its price, the associated risk, the frequency of purchase, and of course, the personality of the buyer.

This perspective on consumer behavior comes from cognitive psychology, which has limited the analysis of emotional implications.

However, studies conducted on *merchandising* show that around 70 percent of decisions are made at the same point of sale, which shows that certain purchases are made in very short periods. This limitation would prevent considering all aspects to make the best decision.

In short, when a person discovers a need and decides to satisfy it, a process of searching for information begins where the opinions of others acquire a certain relevance, especially when there is the necessary degree of trust.

At this point, a new type of consumer appears, which completes an opinion leader's concept. Toffler coined the term in his work *The Third Wave* (1980), where he refers to a new agent of the global village, which is not limited to its role as a consumer but can also provide other goods or services network.

The term's evolution has allowed the integration with other concepts and tendencies until resulting in the conception proposed here.

According to the study carried out by the advertising agency Euro RSCG, *Prosumer Pulse 2005*, "the prosumer is a proactive person, eager for information and opinions, who actively shares his views and experiences with others."

They are people with leadership and persuasiveness who actively live the brand and who want to spread their message because they feel it as their own. This communication ability is what differentiates the consumer as the traditional opinion leader.

Although this new dimension of the concept is somewhat far from the origin of the term, the truth is that the consumer, as described by Toffler, is also a person who anticipates events intending to adapt his offer to the needs of the applicants, seeking mutual benefit.

What differentiates these people from the rest is their ability to adapt to new situations. This flexibility is a characteristic of emotional intelligence.

Emotional intelligence

As we discussed at the beginning of this section, the latest studies on brain activity have discovered the true importance of emotion as a key factor for the human mind's proper functioning. As Damasio points out in his classic work, *The Error of Descartes* (1996), body and mind act as an inseparable set that interacts with the environment.

This allows us to understand that reason may not be as pure as most of us think or wish it was, that emotions and feelings may not be intruders at all in the bastion of reason: they may be entangled in its networks, for the worst and the best.

This accredited Portuguese neurologist demonstrates this fact by studying cases of patients with brain injuries who are unable to lead a normal life despite keeping all their cognitive abilities intact. In short, people have lost certain basic abilities to live in society, including planning time and the future. These skills are not usually measured on intelligence tests.

This very limited view of human intelligence has worried certain psychologists like Goleman, who has proposed a broader approach that includes the study of so-called emotional intelligence. As stated in his work, emotional intelligence is a way of interacting with the world that takes emotions into account and includes impulse control, self-awareness, motivation, enthusiasm, empathy, and mental agility.

Although, as a psychologist, Goleman focuses on knowing how to control human emotions to improve social and personal life, his physiological analysis finds that the functioning of the human brain is not always rational.

This author wonders, "how can we be so rational at one point and so irrational the next." This is explained by his conception of the human mind, made up of two perfectly combined pieces, the rational and the emotional. However, certain events can affect this gear, which could throw the balance to one side.

The emotional mind is characterized by its speed and clairvoyance, which allows us to make decisions at critical moments, a key fact for human evolution. Of course, the emotional brain is influenced by social and cultural contexts. Could this explain impulse buying decisions? Are consumers emotionally intelligent people?

In general, it would be interesting to deepen to what extent the emotional and rational minds work in parallel in the purchase decision process. In other words, Cartesian dualism has had consequences such as a vision of the purchasing decision process focused almost exclusively on the rational mind, an antagonistic approach to advertising strategy, which must choose between rational or emotional axes, when in fact, they are two aspects of the same reality.

The best example of emotional intelligence is the state of flow, which, if we remember as a state that represents the highest degree of control of emotions in the service of performance and learning.

A state in which people are absorbed by complete and undivided attention to what he is doing, and his consciousness merges with his action (Goleman, 2004: 145-146).

In principle, anyone could achieve this maximum degree of emotional control through attention and concentration. The goal is to overcome barriers of attention and focus on work so that we can overcome ourselves.

Saving the distances, the specialists of *one-to-one marketing* try to achieve this maximum attention by personalizing communication and interaction with the user. In short, create a relaxed atmosphere where the brand is founded with leisure and entertainment activities.

Imagine for a moment that someone has entered a website and is so drawn to the site, both for its content and its design, that they forget why they got there. He's fine. He likes what he sees, plays, reads, downloads games… In short, he lives the brand in a relaxed and pleasant environment.

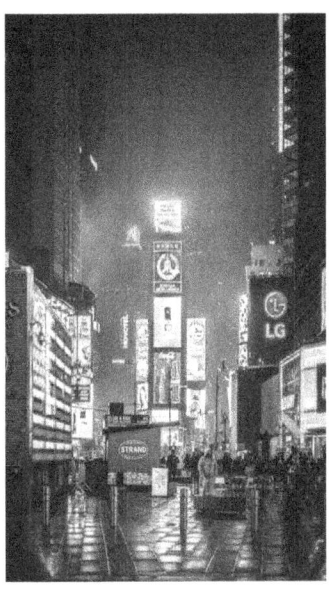

Neuromarketing

Neuroscience is a new discipline that studies the human brain's functioning when it tries to assimilate any stimulus through advanced techniques. Among them, tomography allows us to see how and where the human brain acts in the face of external stimuli.

Therefore, *neuromarketing* supposes the application of the advances of this discipline in the field of *marketing*. According to Braidot, "its purpose is to incorporate knowledge about brain processes to improve the effectiveness of each of the actions that determine the relationship of an organization with its customers."

The latest studies carried out in *neuromarketing* showed that some product preferences, such as the eternal dispute between *Coca-Cola* or *Pepsi,* are more related to the right hemisphere, precisely where the emotion is located.

Scientists at the Baylor School of Medicine in the US have found that the decision between Coca-Cola and Pepsi is not due to their taste but also to the brand's emotional and cultural issues. The experiments' results were surprising since participants who did not know which brand they were drinking activated a different region of the brain than those who did know the brand.

In the first case, the participants opted for Pepsi, and the region activated as the ventromedial prefrontal cortex related to the basic desires in the reward processes. This refers to taste.

On the contrary, when they knew the brand they were drinking, the volunteers leaned for Coca-Cola.

Other parts of the brain related to changes in behavior moved by emotion and affect were activated (hippocampus, midbrain, and dorsolateral prefrontal cortex).

Although it should be noted that the tests were conducted with non-carbonated soft drinks because the scanners do not recognize carbonated drinks.

Although most of the sections consulted on this concept, generally of an informative nature, do not make special mention of the methodological issue, there is an excessive triumphalism in this regard. When they refer to the methodological question, it is superficial or too optimistic.

When a new technique comes to verify what scientists have been trying to decipher for several decades, you must be cautious. Not in vain, advertisers, especially creatives, have been trying for a long time to connect with the most emotional part of human beings. It seems that with the scientific rigor that surrounds this type of discipline, advertisers and designers will have an "infallible" tool to know the effect of your creations.

But they are still experimenting that need a calm reflection on their methodology and their results. Meanwhile, specialized consultancies and advertisers with enough financial capacity to assume the risks have already emerged.

As José Luis León affirms, the function of advertising is to create a climate of trust and closeness with the target audience, leaving aside the more technical and rational aspects, more typical of the business world.

However, advertising, in its search for the prediction of human behavior, has joined forces with research, a field dominated by systematization and rationality: advertising is an excellent territory in which, like no other, they live in conflict with art and science that has always enjoyed their territories, usually mutually exclusive, have been forced to coexist in the advertising universe strangely.

For this reason, *marketing* professionals, closer to research and results from measurement, are very attentive to advances in neuroscience. However, ad creatives have not been surprised by these discoveries, as they test the human brain's complex workings with the results of their campaigns.

However, despite their search for emotional truth, their creative possibilities will be diminished. All this, if finally, the experiments in *neuromarketing* give good results to predict human preferences.

Emotional usability: Kansei engineering

The design has also suffered from this dualism between reason and emotion. Proof of this is the conflict between art and functionality that certain projects of little professionalism generate. From our perspective, both functional and aesthetic values are configurative elements of any design application, from graphic to interactive.

In this sense, we must remember that design, beyond its application to any discipline, tries to communicate messages to a set of people (target audience) with a series of specific characteristics. In this way, Wong refers to the designer's task: A good design is the best visual expression of the essence of something, be it a message or a product. To do it faithfully and effectively, the designer must seek not only for that something to be confirmed.

This can also be applied to website design, which in its obsession with applying usability principles, has neglected other aspects, such as the creativity or personality of some brands in their virtual presence.

Traditionally, the Internet has been considered a cognitive medium, and from this perspective, the accessible and functional website has been created, considering the Internet user as a rational user.

However, sometimes some websites are successful despite not complying with the principles of usability. For this reason, design professionals are reviving an old imported concept of industrial design: *Kansei* engineering.

This discipline, developed in Japan by Mitsuo Nagamachi in the 70s, focuses on studying the quality of an object to produce pleasure when it is used. Design also seeks to apply emotional values to products' production: Can a product express an emotion? Can a car connect emotionally with its audience? To this type of answer, the emotional design or *Kansei* tries to respond.

This Japanese word refers to sensitivity applied to product design.

Eastern culture has traditionally been concerned with the balance between mind and body. And it seems that their products reflect that philosophy that pampers the aesthetics of the product without forgetting its ultimate goal.

Kansei engineering is a method of incorporating emotional variables into product design. A way of systematizing what until now has been considered uncontrollable: emotions. Can the appearance of a product provoke emotions?

Although the use of this term was limited to experts in industrial design, its application to web design has generalized its principles, until it has become a discipline with its characteristics that have even led to usability experts, such as Norman (2005), revised his treatises to incorporate emotional values. This supposes creating a discipline with its entity that receives different names: emotional design, emotional usability, among others.

In summary, we could say that the products with the highest aesthetic value seem easier to use than less attractive ones. Indeed, it is a question of perception because "the emotional system is capable of changing the operational modality of the cognitive system" (Norman, 2005: 34).

Norman explains brain entanglement through three interacting levels of processing: the visceral level, before thought, the behavioral level, which refers to the experience of use. And the reflective level, where understanding, thinking and concentration function mediated by cultural, social, and personal preferences. Each one requires a different design, but they must be considered together if they are satisfied at all levels.

Quick and stereotyped judgments characterize the visceral level. In this sense, the visceral design aims to highlight those attractive physical characteristics at first glance before thought acts. The result could be very basic but eye-catching products with "very intense and bright primary colors."

Regarding the behavioral level, we are especially interested in the physical sensation of the products, the noise of an engine, or the sensation of robustness when closing the door of a Volkswagen brand car.

A study by Millward Brown demonstrated the importance of sensory experiences in branding, which can lead to higher sales. The study's objective was to create an inventory of sensory impressions for a selected set of brands to detect how users experience these sensations and how they can affect their relationship with the brand.

Finally, the reflective design is the most complex as it refers to the meaning we bring to objects, situations, and people around us based on our educational and cultural level. At this level, the brand's image and its positioning in the mind of the consumer works. It is a personal matter that comes from individual experience with the product, so an enriching contact with the brand is essential. At this level, are the brand communities and? Prosumers? Skillful to communicate that experience and recommend the product or service to other people.

Although, as we have pointed out before, the object of desire may not be the product itself, what we imagine ourselves doing with the product, which ultimately inspires us.

Desmet distinguishes between *A-emotions*, that is, those emotions caused by the characteristics of the product (colors, aesthetics, materials) that correspond to the visceral and behavioral levels proposed by Norman; and *R-emotions*, that is, those emotions motivated by what the product represents and inspires (reflective level) that are based on the representation of the product, on what we imagine we will do with it.

Although, from our perspective, we consider that it is a combination, normally, we tend to like a product for its color, texture, and aesthetics, in short for its design, but also because we imagine what we will feel when using it. All this is because the cognitive and emotional levels work in a network, interacting with each other, and modifying our perception. The first, being tangible, has interested the experts in *Kansei more to* find some valid method to incorporate these variables from the beginning of the product design. In this sense, some brands have already incorporated some of these concepts into their design processes, especially the automotive sector, where the differences between benefits hardly exist, making it necessary to distinguish the car by its design, by its brand. Mazda is one of the brands that has put these concepts into practice and has proven its results with the MX5 model, a convertible that has become one of the world's best sellers.

Scientific advances on the human brain's functioning have shown the high involvement of emotions in mental processes. The relationships between the left and right hemispheres explain the complex web of attribution of meanings to what we do, think, or buy. For this reason, brands would have to incorporate all these concepts from product design to *marketing* and communication strategy to manage the entire consumer experience.

Emotional intelligence and the awkward side of web design

Emotional intelligence is described as the ability to generate empathy with others, putting ourselves in their place. Day by day, technology becomes much more humanized. And platforms offer an increasingly personalized user experience.

In this sense, the programming and web design of the different digital products must strive to find a way to have "emotional intelligence" and connect with users.

Twitter celebrated its 10th birthday in March 2016. It was a day of pride for the organization and all of its supporters. It launched a fun heart button/animation to make the day amazing for its users.

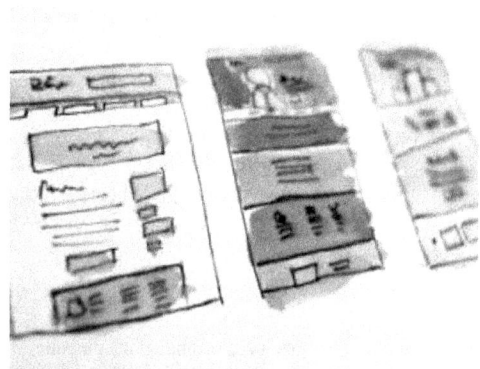

It was amazing, but the animation went way too far as soon as the day ended. Some people didn't care, and others didn't even notice, but there was a hole left behind for those who did. This is not an exaggeration; with confetti, the heart bursts bounce and is cheerful and vibrant. Overall, the boring activities of liking or preferring a tweet made it much more interesting and enjoyable.

Let's talk about the look of hearts vs. stars as well - if you remember, Twitter changed its user interface from stars to hearts in late 2015. "The heart is a universal symbol, a symbol that is far more inclusive," Casey Newton said. Take a look at what the new Heart UI is all about in Twitter's gif. (No, it has not been the same as the confetti explosion since his birthday.)

Since Twitter was involved in increasing interaction for progress, the decision was business-oriented. But how does the heart react adequately to a negative comment? It's not; it's pointless and insensitive. Often a star is worthless, which is exactly why it matters.

Not only is it a Twitter problem, it doesn't have anything to do specifically with Twitter, but it's a perfect example. What if there was a horrible news accident?

By generating more forms of answers, Facebook manages this dilemma. Providing emotionally intelligent responses is still very difficult for a social network, but the acceptance of multiple responses by Facebook is a step forward.

Siri doesn't know how to deal with this either, because we're in it. In critical cases, there are several posts on Siri that do not provide practical support. However, Apple offered useful responses and actions for rape victims and concerns about suicide via a software update in April 2016.

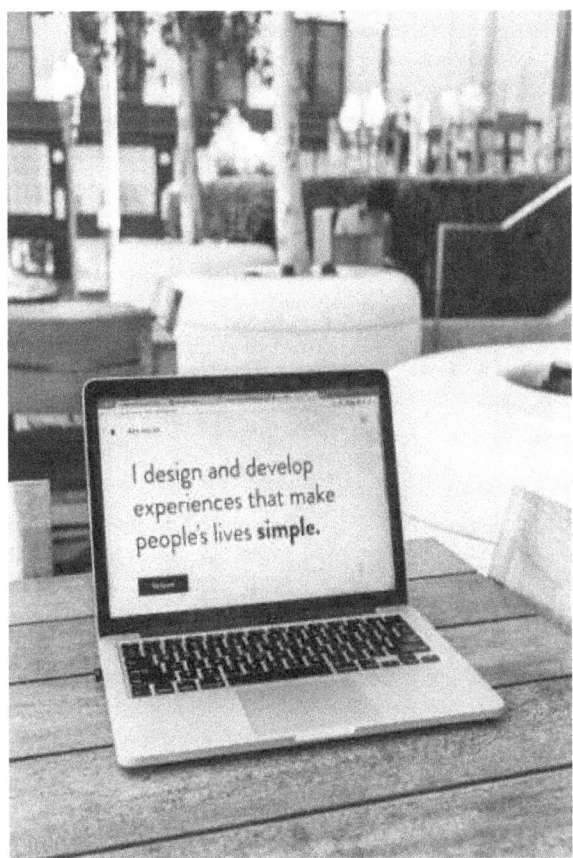

The intelligence of emotions and architecture

Beth Dean wrote an excellent Medium post about traumatic encounters that technology unwittingly brought up. The blog post was inspired by a website that asked her if she knew her deceased mother while trying to verify her identity (it's absolutely nothing compared to making a simple animation). Beth talks about designing from her viewpoint. Emotional intelligence, with. With five traits: self-awareness, self-regulation motivation, empathy, and human ability, she described emotional intelligence.

Knowledge of oneself and self-regulation

Facebook offers a perfect example of self-awareness, asking a user to see advertising based on their conduct. It provides not just a great user experience. It is more important to the user.

As a smart strategy for numbers, Dean explains self-regulation. Just because the numbers are going up doesn't mean that it's all right. A website that spammed the contacts of a user to improve their interaction was the example you used. Of course, interaction improved, but as soon as the customer realized that they approached their contacts reluctantly, trust in the business decreased. That is why you see the message, "we will not publish on your behalf" when you visit a site via a social network such as Facebook, Google, or Twitter.

Motivation, empathy, and talents of humans

It is a little difficult to understand motivation, but it comes down to the users' perspective and their particular context. It's about trying to make the target audience understand and not disrespect others who are not. You don't want your app to feel rejected by anyone. A little modesty can go a long way when it comes to empathy.

That leaves us with the abilities of humans. When it comes to tech, what a fascinating concept to speak about, don't you think? Human abilities apply to the general tone used by the product and the external environment it projects. It is about useful, but also a suitable material.

We need to be mindful of these aspects to develop and program systems and goods for a more human experience.

It is possible to see empathy and emotional intelligence as software seeks to be inclusive. In her post, Dean states that she is now very used to "tech personalities" and recognizes that software is designed for the majority. To include all possible scenarios, the most impressive software can, therefore, be developed.

Chapter 6: The Black Dog

Sir Winston Churchill, the former Prime Minister of the United Kingdom who steered the country towards Second World War victory, struggled from depression. He metaphorically called his depressive state, "a black dog."

Such a metaphor is widely discussed over the internet. In the context of this chapter, we are going to shed light on psychological techniques and proposals on "leashing the blackdog." In other words, controlling and minuting symptoms of depression.

We start by exploring different theories that explain depression.

The theory of response styles: this is how it explains depression

This theory, proposed by Susan Nolen-Hoeksema, talks about the nexus between depression and rumination.

In Psychology, many theories have been proposed to explain the origin and maintenance of depression: learning, cognitive, social theories.

Today **we will learn about Susan Nolen-Hoeksema's theory of response styles**, a cognitive-social model that alludes to the subject's reflective style to explain the emergence of depressive disorder.

Some people turn things around a lot, even going into a loop and doing absolutely nothing to remedy their problems. We are talking about a ruminative thinking style. But how is this style of thinking related to depression? We will see it next.

Theory of response styles

The theory of response styles is a theory encompassed within cognitive-social models **proposed by Susan Nolen-Hoeksema (1991, 2000), an American psychologist** and professor at Yale University.

When Nolen-Hoeksema began the studies on ruminative style, she found that **ruminative thinking and depression** did not show significant differences between girls and boys during childhood.

However, from adolescence, both elements' presence was double in the case of women, remaining constant during the rest of their life cycle (Nolen-Hoeksema, 1991).

The author alluded to the factors that determine the course of depression. According to the theory of response styles, **how the subject responds to the first symptoms of depression** influences its duration and severity.

The theory does not explain the origin of depression, if not its maintenance and exacerbation.

The ruminative style in depression

Ruminative style or rumination are repetitive ideas about sadness itself, its causes, and possible consequences. It is a predictor of some psychopathologies and is linked to depression, as Nolen-Hoeksema suggests.

Also, it can be considered a type of coping strategy in situations of stress and discomfort. However, it is considered dysfunctional and maladaptive, **reaching consequences as serious as suicide, in extreme cases**.

According to the theory of response styles, once you have depression, focusing attention on the symptoms and their implications without doing anything to alleviate them (exhibiting a ruminative response style) will maintain or exacerbate depressive symptoms.

This style is the opposite of an active style based on distraction or problem solving, which would be functional and adaptive.

Numerous experimental and field studies support the theory of S. Nolen-Hoeksema and affirm that a ruminant response style in a subject **increases the probability that a depressed mood will intensify**, even becoming a depressive disorder.

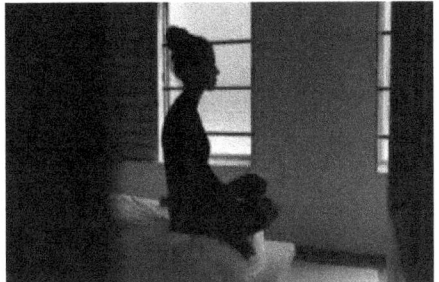

Ruminant style mechanisms

The theory of response styles raises a series of **mechanisms that explain the negative effects of the ruminant style**, which are the following:

1. Vicious circles

Vicious cycles occur between depressed mood and the **negative cognitions** associated with depression.

These two elements influence each other and feedback, causing depression to become chronic and accentuate.

2. Decrease in the generation of effective solutions

The generation of solutions aimed at solving basic problems is practically nil.

Thus, **the subject does nothing or practically nothing to solve his situation**. He simply "turns around" what is happening to him, without reaching any conclusion or putting any solution into practice.

3. Interference with instrumental behaviors

The ruminative style negatively interferes with instrumental behaviors that would provide reinforcement and a sense of control to the subject.

In other words, rumination will hinder the generation and implementation of such behaviors; in this way, the subject **will enter a state of helplessness and hopelessness** that will lead him to "do nothing."

4. Weakening of social support

Social support is reduced or disappears due to the patient's behavior, which **provokes criticism and rejection among his family and friends**.

Origin of the ruminant style

The ruminative style that the theory of response styles raises is originated by learning in childhood, **through modeling and certain socialization practices** that do not provide a more adaptive repertoire of behaviors.

Results in experimental studies

Ruminative responses have been investigated in experimental studies, and the following effects of having a ruminative thinking style have been observed:

- Increase in negative and global attributions.
- Increased accessibility of negative memories.
- **Pessimism and biased negative interpretations**.
- Generation of poorer interpersonal solutions.

On the other hand, it has also been seen how rumination can be a predictor of anxiety symptoms, in addition to depressive symptoms, in individuals with or without pre-existing depression.

The link between depression and perfectionism

How is the tendency to be perfectionism and the probability of having depression associated with each other?

Depression is a very common alteration of mental health, and this is, among other things, because this emotional state is not reached by a single route but by several.

Depression is sometimes discussed with the assumption that it is simply an illness and that, as such, it is caused solely by biological complications in the person's body. Still, the truth is that personality traits and lifestyle habits can explain a good part of our propensity to develop this disorder.

This section will focus on **the relationship between depression and perfectionism**, two highly studied psychological phenomena in which points of interconnection have been seen. And it is that many times we tend to associate perfectionism with a positive and useful aspect of the personality (and to a certain extent). In excess, it can compromise our mental health in different ways.

What do these concepts mean in psychology?

First, let's clarify the concepts that we are going to talk about. Depression is **a mood disorder characterized by a lack of energy and motivation, low expectations, and a state of sadness or anguish** that makes it very difficult to enjoy life's pleasant experiences (a vacation, dinner at a good restaurant, etc.). As a psychological disorder, its presence not only implies discomfort but also negatively affects the quality of life of those who suffer it and increases the risk of suicide.

On the other hand, **perfectionism is scrupulous when evaluating the product of our actions**. This means that we pay attention to the need to do things right and that the idea of creating something with one or more imperfections causes us discomfort.

The relationship between depression and degree of perfectionism

Different ways are tending to a high degree of perfectionism are associated with the probability of having depression. Here we will see several of them, although one thing must be borne in mind: being a perfectionist does not mean that this trait will generate a depressive disorder. Sometimes what happens is that what leads us to develop perfectionism also leads us to develop depression.

Differences between types of perfectionism

First, a distinction must be made between two types of perfectionism: **perfectionist aspirations and perfectionist concerns**. The second of these forms of perfectionism consists of the propensity to worry about the possibility of doing things wrong, the anticipation of failure if we do not pay much attention to what we are doing, and the obsession with avoiding a bad result. However, the first has to do with wanting to be the best version of ourselves and giving importance to doing things in the best possible way.

In this way, perfectionist aspirations are linked to a higher risk of manifesting stress and anxiety problems. In contrast, perfectionist concerns are associated with the risk of suffering from depression.

Those who adopt this type of perfectionism focus their attention on the negative aspect of their skills and abilities and spend a lot of time anticipating and imagining poor results in what they do. The latter fosters emotional fatigue and the inability to enjoy.

Of course, we must not forget that those who follow the path of perfectionist aspirations are not exempt from presenting a greater risk of having depression because **anxiety overlaps a lot with mood disorders**.

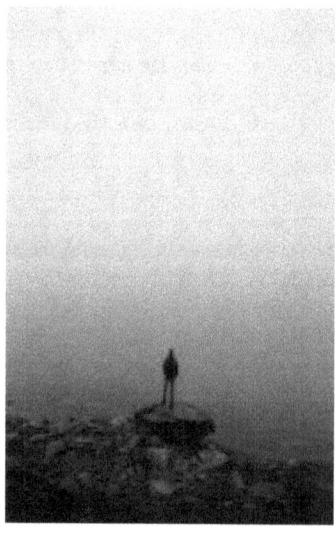

Eating disorders

It has been seen that the risk of developing eating disorders, such as anorexia nervosa or bulimia, is associated with a tendency to high or very high perfectionism, which makes sense considering that the discomfort comes from thinking in imperfections in behavior and physical condition.

This is relevant because, **as is often the case with treatable psychological disorders in therapy, having developed one makes it more likely that we will develop another**, and depression is at the top of the list of possible risks.

Work addiction

The tendency to work too much, closely linked to perfectionism, is related to the risk of developing depression in the medium and long term.

There are different explanations for why this happens. One of them is that, as "workaholics" transform their work environment into the main focus of interest in their lives, **little by little, they are cutting off their links with other sources of satisfaction and social life.**

When they find that they cannot keep up with that rhythm of concentration and effort, they find themselves alone and socially isolated, with no stimulating hobbies and, in general, no reason to stop directing 100% of their attention to their work performance. This is the point where depression lands.

On the other hand, the extreme concern to produce and do everything well that causes addiction to work is also linked to lack of sleep, which is most linked to depression if the nervous system does not have time to recover. In contrast, we sleep—the chances of developing mood disorders skyrocket.

How to get out of depression? Tips and effective treatments

What to do when we are going through a time of depression? Going to psychotherapy requires a commitment and effort to change the part of the patient with his reality.

Healthy changes in behavior cannot be made without willpower, effort, and motivation. But ... **How is it possible to be motivated when I feel depressed?** Next, I will indicate some concepts that will help you identify depressive symptoms and tools to combat them.

What to do about depressive symptoms

First of all, it is important to know that to the extent that we are focused on the negative aspects of any aspect of our life. **As we focus on the bad things that happen to us, we take our attention away from the good and positive things.** This ends up becoming a habit for your mind. When depression has been in you for a long time, this connection is so important that you practically cancel out everything positive.

It is sabotage of everything that can be good since your brain automatically looks for something negative to replace it since you have somehow programmed it for that.

One thing I warn you about is that **it is not possible to change the connection and the focus of attention from one day to the next**. But you can start by identifying the things you used to like to do and now don't. As you identify the "negative programming" that you have built with **constant negative thoughts** and behaviors that reinforce it, you will plan new programming with a more positive approach.

Attention is the ability to concentrate on a particular stimulus that we have selected from among others.

To attend to a stimulus, it is necessary to neglect others. For example, when watching an interesting movie, we turn our attention away from our mobile phone or other things around us. Depression is a disease that collapses people's attention span, and thought processes respond to an involuntary demand for attention.

Therefore, it is important to take stock of the things that are given importance. With therapeutic help, you will be able to change the focus of attention characteristic of depression to recover motivation, illusion, and moments of well-being gradually.

Depressive behaviors take time to settle in your body and mind. It is very likely that this disease's trigger comes from unpleasant experiences or that you do not know exactly its origin. The important thing is to analyze to what extent you have come to program your mind so that the moment of sadness remains established in you.

Why do you get depressed?

Depression is a way to connect with the world and face life. It allows us to constantly remember what could not be done, our defects, what we lack, etc. The difference with a positive connection is looking at all these aspects and, in turn, looking for a solution. Therefore, we would be connecting with things that can be changed. We would begin to change the focus of attention with a balance of thoughts that are not negative.

It is normal, natural, and healthy for you to feel sad at different times in your life.

But when that sadness changes the environment and stops doing the things you like, abandon projects, and despair grows in you, sadness becomes a pathology, so self-evaluation is important to avoid that pathological sadness. Depression continues to take away your moments of enjoyment and well-being.

Get out of depression

It is not easy, but it is possible. If you gradually build a stimulating environment around you, focusing your attention on the positive that you have, and planning activities that allow you to connect with the things you like, things will fall into place.

The depression will fade over time. You must know that, just as depression takes time to set in, you have to be constant in the implementation of positive behaviors to change your perception of the environment. If you don't, depression will take more and more space in your mind and body, going through different degrees of mild, moderate, and severe.

Even in chronic cases, other mental disorders may be associated with depression due to the magnitude of the lack of control of your habits and thoughts. Therefore, it is important to make changes in thought and behavior processes that can influence the creation of an environment that promotes greater well-being and growth.

Depression is a disease that all people can suffer from. Unlike sadness, it is a lifestyle that is adopted with negative habits that are repeated daily, added to the thoughts that allow depression to persist.

You must go to a mental health professional since the techniques described above are only useful strategies that, by themselves, do not replace what a psychotherapy process is. The psychologist will intervene individually in your case to have the necessary tools to deal with your depression effectively.

Behavioral Activation as a therapy against depression

Jacobson (1996) called Behavioral Activation (AC) to the programming of activities, applied together with cognitive intervention techniques, which improve any behavioral deficit or excess in the person.

It is **a therapy aimed at treating depression** and understands the behaviors of the person who suffers from it as a symptom and as part of the essence and maintenance of the disorder.

What is Behavioral Activation?

Among the symptoms of depression, one of the most characteristic is inaction, which is part of a vicious circle in which the person suffering from it is immersed: the lack of activity affects the mood. In the same way, a depressed mood produces a lack of activity. This relationship is the epicenter of the Behavioral Activation proposal, which considers some types of depression as elaborate forms of avoidance.

This therapy's objective, framed within the third generation therapies of the cognitive-behavioral current, and which is itself a therapy itself, is that depressed patients can organize their lives and change their environment to **reestablish their relationship with sources of stimulus that provide positive reinforcement for them**.

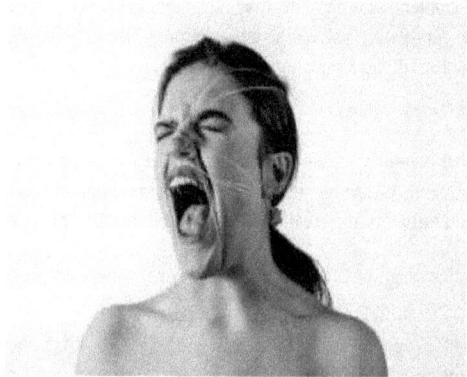

Some of the interventions with behavioral activation methods aimed at reducing depressive symptoms are the prioritization of tasks, the programming of vital objectives, the reinforcement of social contact behaviors, and the performance of rewarding activities.

How does it work?

The therapy is mainly based on **prescribing activities to break the dynamics of inactivity**. To be effective, especially at the beginning, it is necessary that the programming includes easy, rewarding activities (not only pleasant, since we look for activities that are satisfactory and require effort) gradual and that are very well planned, then, especially at the beginning of the program, but it is also easy that difficulties arise for its realization.

Current meta-analytic reviews (Cuijpers, van Straten & Warmer-dam, 2007) and experimental studies in which different therapeutic approaches have been compared - antidepressant medication, cognitive therapy, and behavioral activation therapy— (Dimidjian et al., 2006) have revealed that **purely behavioral interventions are sufficient** for an efficient and effective approach to depressive conditions.

Its advantages

Some of the advantages of Behavioral Activation programs are as follows.

Has shown extensive scientific evidence: Compared with pharmacological therapy, it has obtained comparable results and **a higher percentage of remission in the subjects and adherence to treatment**.

It is a simple treatment to apply: Compared to other proposals, it does not require so many steps.

Does not require modification of thoughts, whose procedure is more complex: The data suggest that the application of the behavioral components by themselves **achieves the same result as full cognitive therapy**.

In short, Behavioral Activation is therapy with strong empirical support, which offers a new treatment opportunity for people suffering from depression.

The four coping strategies for depression

Various initiatives to combat the damaging effects of depression and improve quality of life.

Depression is characterized by **maintaining a state of deep sadness** for **more than two weeks, often without knowing why.** Unlike sadness as an emotion, which is transitory and generally caused by something perceived as negative for the person.

To this is added **an absence of pleasure and lack of motivation for any activity**. An alteration in appetite and weight is experienced, since sometimes there is a loss of them, while in some cases the person shows an excessive appetite.

In the same way, **sleep is also affected** by insomnia or excess non-restorative sleep. The person presents fatigue or loss of energy, showing dejection in his face and lack of care in his person, in addition to walking, moving, and speaking slowly.

However, the characteristics of depression are not limited to physical alterations such as those just shown, since the person also experiences feelings of worthlessness and guilt for unimportant things, as if it were a nuisance for the people around him. Inevitably, limitations in mental capacity appear. That is, thinking slows down, and attention and concentration decrease.

Finally, **thoughts of hopelessness appear**, showing apathy towards life, so the person thinks of death as a remedy. According to the WHO, each year, about 800,000 people commit suicide, which represents the second cause of death among young people between 15 and 29 years old.

Coping strategies for depression

What to do when a friend or family member suffers from depression? Let's see.

1. Acknowledge your suffering

First, you need to listen to and acknowledge their suffering. Suddenly, you usually try to encourage the person using phrases such as: "Courage! Don't be sad", "Don't cry anymore," causing guilt and frustration, since it is not something that depends on the person how to feel.

Instead, **when their feelings are validated, and empathy is shown, we become companions**.

2. Don't feed your sadness

It is not about reinforcing their condition by fostering self-compassion or incapacitating the person but treating them as someone going through a difficult time. Likewise, it helps the family member keep busy **with walks, entertainment, small jobs, etc.**

3. Taking any suggestion or threat of suicide seriously

A serious mistake is made when signals of this type are ignored, as the person may be giving a warning. **The best thing to do is to keep an eye on the person with depression**, not leaving them alone for a long time.

4. Seek professional help

At this point, it is very common to only resort to medication. However, despite being useful, it only reduces the symptoms but does not solve depression. So, it is common to find people under drug treatment dealing with depression for a long time: months or more than a year.

Also, the person on antidepressant medication does not begin to notice the medication's effects until two to three weeks after starting treatment. So, **the most advisable thing is to start a psychotherapeutic process to work in the required areas**.

Tips to prevent this mental disorder

These are some recommendations to apply on a day-to-day basis.

1. Do aerobic physical exercise

The chemical and hormonal balance produced by drugs can also be achieved or supplemented with sports and physical activity.

Fatigue is a source of health and good humor since **this kind of exercise produces serotonin**, which is a neurotransmitter related to feelings of pleasure and well-being. It also promotes a state of mental peace, reduces levels of daily stress, and improves self-esteem.

These benefits are better than the most effective antidepressant, and sadly, they are least followed.

2. Avoid isolation

A study (Nolen-Hoaksema and Morrow, 1991) carried out in San Francisco (USA) showed that **isolation favors depressive emotions and thoughts**. It is advisable to have a support network, such as friends or family.

3. Stay busy or busy

Whether outdoors or at home, look for an occupation; that way, the activities will help keep your mind off the thoughts that accentuate depression.

4. Seek professional help

If these tips are not enough, **the psychologist's help will always be the best option to get out of depression**. Proper psychotherapy can achieve the desired results.

Depression is a complex problem, so the recovery process is often slow, so that patience is required from both the affected person and those around him. Although depression often requires psychological intervention, self-help strategies are beneficial for psychological treatment and even prevention.

The benefits of having psychotherapeutic and psychiatric care

What are the aspects of the psychiatric intervention that reinforce psychotherapeutic support?

It is often assumed that psychotherapy and psychiatric treatments are two opposing ways of working, competing with each other to improve people's well-being, and ensure their mental health.

However, the truth is that the idea that these two forms of intervention in patients are mutually exclusive does not make sense. Nowadays, it is known that combining both things helps a lot when treating certain disorders.

In this section, we will see how **having both psychotherapy and psychiatric support** benefits patients and why, in some cases, it is the most recommended option.

Differences between the work of the psychologist and the psychiatrist

First of all, let's see what the aspects in which psychiatric intervention and psychotherapy differ are.

Psychotherapy is a concept applied to the need to solve a wide variety of **problems related to behavior, thinking, and emotions**.

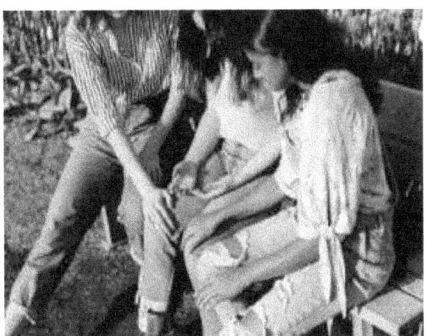

This implies that it is not limited to offering services to people who have developed a psychological disorder; for example, some people go to psychological therapy to stop having low self-esteem, improve their communication or social skills, or even better manage couple arguments.

Furthermore, psychotherapy is fundamentally a learning process: patients learn both theoretical aspects of what is happening to them and how they can solve it and practical ones, about how to overcome this problem by adopting new habits and styles of thinking.

On the other hand, **psychiatry proposes resources from the world of medicine** since, after all, psychiatrists are doctors specialized in mental health. For this reason, they work in cases in which there is (or may exist) a disorder, so they care for people whose quality of life is being significantly affected regularly.

It is very common for the use of psychotropic drugs to be proposed, although always strictly following their instructions, since these products may have side effects to be taken into account.

The benefits of having psychiatric and psychotherapeutic support

These are the main advantages of having help in both ways combined, psychotherapeutic, and psychiatric.

1. Psychiatric support helps meet the goals of psychotherapy

Sometimes the symptoms of the disorder that affect the patient are so intense that it makes it difficult for them to reach the goals set in psychotherapy or even prevent them from concentrating and understanding what to do.

In these cases, the use of drugs or other psychiatric tools can allow **you to reach a point where the discomfort is reduced enough to get involved with the tasks associated with psychological therapy**, and from there, continue to improve.

2. Psychiatric intervention helps a lot in crisis

In acute discomfort cases, in which it is a priority to make the discomfort go down as soon as possible, psychiatric intervention may offer somewhat faster ways of action than psychotherapy. And once that phase has passed, **having a psychiatric professional allows you to detect in time the signs that another crisis of this type could arise**.

3. The combined use of both interventions intensifies their effects

On many occasions in which there are severe psychiatric or psychological disorders, the effects of psychotherapy and psychiatric intervention **are mutually reinforcing in terms of patient improvement consistency**. They feel better and more consistently.

4. Psychological support helps to commit to both therapies

Finally, psychotherapy predisposes patients to commit more to their process of improvement and recovery of well-being. Its **effects extend beyond the motivation to continue going to the psychologist** (as long as it is necessary) and include the psychiatric route's commitment.

You are loved. You are needed. You are important. And you matter. That is all this time around from me and Oscar. We hope to catch you soon with another entry. Wear a mask.

EMOTIONAL DETOX TO REWIRE YOUR BRAIN TO SUCCESS

Subconscious Mind to Conquer Negative Thinking, Learn the Law of Attraction Manifestation, Unleashing the Power Within Because Failure Is Not an Option

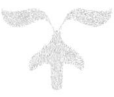

Contents

Chapter I: Defining Negativity — 1

Chapter II: Negativity and Us — 26

Chapter III: The Negativity Bias — 50

Chapter IV: Mind and the Unexpected Stimuli — 69

Chapter V: Positivity As An Imposition — 89

Chapter VI: Theories of Positivity and The Law of Attraction — 108

Homestretch — 141

Chapter I: Defining Negativity

Thinking Thoughts

Have you ever wondered how the thought process functions in our minds? How does the human brain develop to think thoughts, and what function does it serve?

Ever since we are born, and even before that, our minds are constantly thinking. We are performing a function that is innate of the human being. Although we are all born with the ability to think, focused work is necessary for thinking, so that it reaches higher and higher levels of development and is not limited to an automatic function. Otherwise, we would have little or no awareness.

Perkins, in 1998, explains that the minds of young children develop in a culture of thought so that reaching youth and adults, they can be vigilant and cope with complex situations. Such situations include organizing time and establishing a good strategy to take on life, to understand the point of view of another person, be critical of a view, find sideways when a situation appears to have no way out, and detect and deal with unfounded rumors.

Research carried out by the Project Zero team establishes that most of the people have undeveloped thinking skills, attitudes and alerts. They are passively indifferent to thought-provoking circumstances. They are insensitive to signals that invite reflection. They do not cultivate attitudes of deep thought, such as: questioning the evidence, go beyond the obvious, see the hidden side of situations, think differently at least for time and seize all thought-provoking opportunities.

For this reason, children and young people must learn these attitudes, skills and alerts that are promoters of the thought, but they cannot develop spontaneously.

One of the reasons we are not aware of our thoughts is that, luckily or unfortunately, our thoughts are not perceptible to the people around us. And many sometimes, the situations that cause them are also imperceptible.

In the educational field, the possibility of capturing the learning object with our senses facilitates much the process. For example, for a child who is learning to write, visualizing the different lyrics helps you to reproduce them.

For a high school student who is studying the cell, if they have the opportunity to look at a cell under a microscope, more easily a mental image and that said image collaborates with the construction of concepts, for a student learning to play a piece of music on an instrument by listening to the performance.

From an experienced musician, you get an idea about the cadence in which you have to work. At the learning process greatly affect perceptions: The observation of the learning objectives of:

The thought is invisible. In most cases, the thought remains under the hood, inside the wonderful engine of our mind. Fortunately, neither the thought nor opportunities to think must necessarily be invisible as frequently they are.

Directly or indirectly, it allows us to imitate, reproduce, evoke, adapt and transform that perception and to build our knowledge, a knowledge that has a personal mark. The problem arises when the object of learning is thought itself, because the object of study is invisible, at least in the first instance, and the circumstances that provoke it.

Everything "Negativity"

My girlfriend is an incredible visual artist and illustrator. Trust me, one of the best I have ever seen, and I have an art school background. These days she is running an active Instagram Creator profile, displaying her art and building up her social media presence as an artist. Now she is temperamental over the sluggish journey of building her profile from zilch to successful.

To top it off, she recently followed a famed artist: a blue tick Instagram prodigy whose timeline offers a magnanimous visual experience. If you are an artist, you want to be them. This artist started a trend and called up other artists on Instagram to follow suit. The trend translated into a mega-successful hashtag and followed posts in an abundance of thousands.

Of course, my sweetheart was tempted to join the bandwagon. Because she eyed a significant opportunity to grow, garner more engagement and possibly be followed, viewed, or reposted by the originator of the trend. 24 hours later, I find her more excited than she has ever been in 2020. She had posted what she made as part of the big trend and anticipated to blow up – in a positive way, of course.

Next thing I know is receiving a chain of text messages as I was walking to my Uber on my way back home, later that day. Turns out; she did not receive enough engagement as much as she had thought she would. She had scanned the profile of the artist who started the trend, constantly brooding over the mentions of other artists in their stories. Other artists were not even that good, or so I have been told.

Two hours had passed, and there was absolute silence. In her room. On her Instagram. And on the profile of that artist. Reposts and shares in stories had stopped. It felt like the ship has sailed, and we were late to arrive on the dock.

By this time, she was convinced that she was not good enough, that her work failed to make an impression. I found myself scrambling to take her out of those thoughts by constantly reminding her of the excellence she pulled off on that Procreate canvas on iPad. I wanted to scream on top of my lungs so that the likes of Sandro Botticelli could hear and agree with me.

But she was not having it this time. She showed me the hundreds of profiles that had been shared and reached better engagement. She was adamant that she was no good enough. An hour went by, and she was still dissecting what went wrong, actively criticizing her art, and just plainly putting out aspects which did not fit about her work.

As a result, I found herself practicing other styles. She Googled a ton of styles which were very different from hers and began practicing. If she was Renaissance, she was trying the world of Manga now. And it was a recipe for disaster.

The night went past, and we woke up to the same conversation and her sulking morning face. She still looked pretty, to be honest. But it was the dawn of sadness. She once again checked Instagram but all to no avail. Even if there was a beacon of hope, it had gone past now.

 An hour later in the shower, I found myself stuck in thoughts of how to turn around the situation? Maybe get her paid project of growing on Instagram? I was putting pieces back into place when I heard loud knocks on the bathroom door. Of course, I recognized that pattern of knocks.

Next thing I know, she brandished into the bathroom and drew my curtain as if I was Venus on the canvas of our friend Boticelli's "Mars and Venus". I thought Oscar (my dog) had puked again. But it was her iPhone and my distorted vision trying to figure out what she was showing me.

So, good news, the artist had shared her work, liked it, and commented on the post. She was over the moon and I tell you what, he well admired her work. Reflecting upon this personal anecdote, I came to wonder how our cognitive patterns work and to what extent is the human brain susceptible to negative thoughts.

Never again did I find her talking about changing her style or being hyper-critical of her work.

Without defining the term "negativity", we could all find around us a clear example or several, of a negative person. The person that comes to mind is the one who always sees the "glass half empty", who never ends up being happy with anything and when their circumstances change, and it seems that everything will get better, they tell us that they were actually better off before. It can be exhausting for us to listen to it, but it is that person who has the worst time. Their life is done.

There are many types of negative people. Some only want to complain, without listening or attending to possible solutions. The competitors in "the long-distance race of negativity", those who are always going to be worse off than you, because they have the worst luck or because what happened to them was more serious.

And others are the "chronic" negatives, those who are continually thinking about their bad luck, their problems, their unfair life situation, and for whom no relief is enough.

And it is easy to fall into the well of negativity. All of us sometimes put ourselves in the role of victim, complaining without seeking a solution. The psychologist Stephen Karpman developed in 1968 what he called the "Dramatic Triangle."

In it, he explains that many times we enter this role of the victim because it has been the position that we had or chose to survive in our environment, where there were also *rescuers* (who even helped and succor without being asked for help) and *persecutors* (always looking for a victim to reproach, accuse or punish). But even if it is our usual way of functioning, and in fact, it seems to work, it is not a healthy coping mechanism.

Neuropsychologists have investigated negativity and studies claim that, since our brain works through neural networks, if we have repetitive thoughts about something, in particular, it learns to "activate" the same neurons with thoughts, feelings or sensations that are similar.

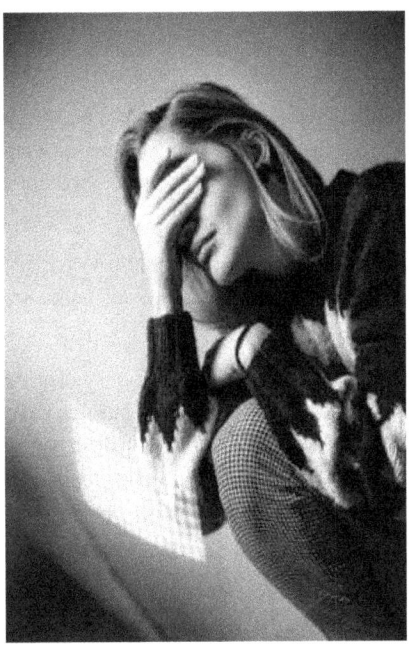

In other words, if we always maintain negative or victimizing ideas, our minds will find it easier to access these networks when we find ourselves in similar situations.

For example, if I trip and my cell phone breaks, if I'm always thinking about my bad luck, my brain will first activate a thought of the type "why does it always happen to me!", And not the type "well, it was so old that I was going to have to change it soon". It means that our negativity makes us more and more negative.

The so-called positive psychology alerts us that the human mind has an irrepressible fondness for the negative. Begun in the 1990s by Martin Seligman and continued by the unpronounceable Mihaly Csikszentmihalyi, and very enlightening Jonathan Haidt, it focuses on the scientific study of psychological wellbeing and several positive aspects from creativity and humor to wisdom or happiness itself.

This branch of psychology is the counterpoint of a long history focused on the study of the neuronal bases – and the possible remedies – of depression, anxiety, stress and other demons and mental pathologies. It seeks to understand and promote positivity in the face of the realization that the bad and threatening runs freely through the mind and is stronger than the good. This principle called the negativity bias, conditions our lives for good and bad.

We will get to negativity bias later in more detail. But for now, the negativity bias may seem like a biological drag. It makes perfect evolutionary sense. Automatic cerebral hyperresponsiveness (faster than conscious decision-making) is what allows us to save our lives against any potential threat. However, they are often false alarms (for example, when we jump in the armchair before the unexpected appearance in a movie of a knife or a snake, or we change the sidewalk because a stranger approaches at night).

The brain lacks a similar system to react to what is good and pleasant because life is not about it. The fact that the negative prevails over the positive in mind is what makes the pain of an economic loss greater than the pleasure of a gain and that the emotions that bad news provokes are stronger.

The Swedish epidemiologist Hans Rosling, famous for his spectacular TED talks with statistics on the progress of countries, has studied for decades the unfounded negative view that Westerners have of the so-called developing world.

The common people believe that in the world there are more violent deaths, fewer girls in school, lower vaccination rates, less access to electricity and the Internet, more species in danger of extinction ... than there really are. And he attributes this instinct of negativity, as he calls it, to the forgetfulness about our past, to the feeling that while things are bad, it is inhumane to recognize that they improve, and the distorted image transmitted by the media and activists.

Rosling's negativity instinct and the negativity bias of positive psychologists refer to the same recent finding in neuroscience. Behind this scientific knowledge, there is certainly whole *pop* psychology that can distort things and extract self-help pills with a more or less scientific basis, but this does not invalidate the proven existence of this quick, tenacious and natural human response to bad and the worst news.

As with everything human, there is great variability between people on the optimism-pessimism scale, which has a strong genetic basis (this is what Jonathan Haidt calls the "cortical lottery", alluding to the frontal cortex of the brain). In these times of pandemic, we can clearly appreciate not only to what extent the negativity bias is present but also the variability of responses between people.

Cycles of Negative Thinking

There are only two types of thoughts, negative and positive. Both work through a cycle that feeds them, and as this progress or happens, it will gain more power. As it feeds on negative energy, it takes on more strength, and the human host is the one who allows it to continue its cycle because it is the mind that generates the thoughts.

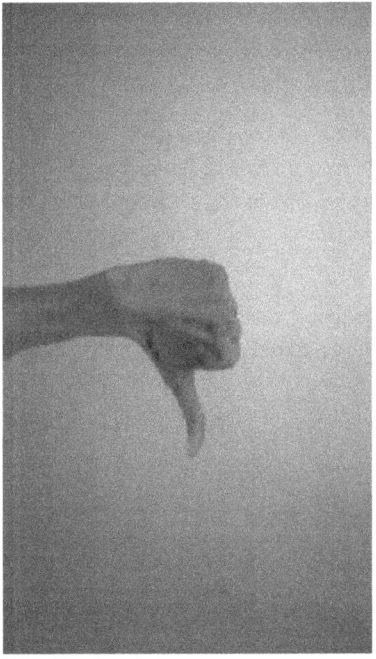

If we think about negative things before the "X" situation, what will be the result of this? Well, without a doubt, we are going to obtain negative results, because we program our minds to obtain them. If we see motivation as an unattainable element, we will not get very far, and we will always be a failure in a difficult situation. Perhaps we focus on the error, on what they will say, on our fears, etc. And we allow them to rule us instead of us ruling them.

A psychology study revealed that the average person has around 4,000 thoughts a day and of those thoughts, 31% are negative thoughts, and the rest are repetitive thoughts. The vast majority of people are trapped in a negative thinking cycle with no idea that it is possible to break out of this cycle.

But for what reason does it seem that our brains evolved to make us think this way?

Negative thinking and repetitive thinking make sense from the perspective of biological evolution, as our ancestors needed this repetitive thinking to deal with the routine activities of every day and negative thinking was just a way to be constantly on the lookout for predators or natural catastrophes.

Your great, great, great, great, great, great, grandfather decided it was best to finish eating the wild boar he had hunted before wolves started to linger around him.

The brain is designed to produce beta waves under survival conditions, but beta waves are the waves that characterize thoughts of fear or stress. Fear was what helped our ancestors survive. Fear is what helped your great – let's just go with it – grandfather live to fight wolves another day.

Although we are no longer living in the jungle trying to escape predators, our brain continues to function as if we still lived in those conditions.

When we wake up in the morning, our brain has been in theta and delta while we were sleeping, but suddenly, it automatically switches to beta. We start to worry because we are already late, we start to stress about everything we have to do that day or for the presentation that we must do in a few hours. We start to worry, and this evolution mechanism that was previously used to detect a predator is activated.

Before leaving the house, our brain is flooded with anxious thoughts. These types of thoughts, or what is called "the brain of the caveman", has a very negative effect on our body.

Thoughts Are Things

In a study of 68,222 adults, anxious thoughts were found to increase the chance of death by 20%.

The same ability that helped our ancestors survive is what is killing many people today. Our mind has become a threat to our survival.

Our mind is like a dark room where photographs are developed. It is the secret place where our external life unfolds.

What we are is not our name, or our physical appearance, or how we dress, or our family, or the car we drive or the place where we live. What we are, are the beliefs that take shape in this dark room.

Our subconscious mind is totally neutral and does not judge whether a habit or belief is good or bad. For this reason, it is normal for us to constantly be surprised to discover all the negative beliefs or images that we have in this mind, which are expressed in our daily experiences over and over again. Rarely something happens to us that we have not created in our mind.

To change our world, we must change what is in this dark room. If you accept this concept of the subconscious mind as a dark room, you will realize that changing your life does not have to be a difficult process. Rather, it is just changing the images that are being revealed in this dark room.

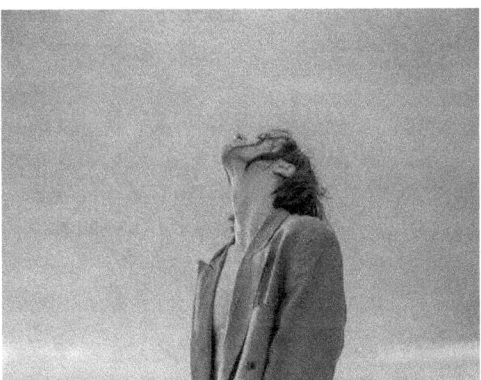

You will be surprised to know that all the beliefs and tendencies that you learned and adopted in your childhood are the images that have the most power and influence in your current life.

All of us have these images that were created by beliefs and ideas, which we have completely forgotten, but are still hidden in the depths of our minds. Knowing this shows you the importance of choosing your thoughts and mental images carefully.

For example, if you have the belief that if someone next to you sneezes you will get sick, then that fear becomes the movement of your mind that creates your expectation and the next time someone next to you sneezes, you will get sick.

On the other hand, where do you think miracle cures come from? They also come from the subconscious mind.

If you fill this dark room with truths, your external world will be the reflection of these internal images that express a truth.

The subconscious mind accepts these truths and acts to instantly heal your body. And not only healings, but wealth creation also occurs in the subconscious mind, and the key is to make the subconscious rich before you can see abundance in your life.

Illness and health are basically the results of our most dominant mental and spiritual states.

An emotional shock, a mind full of fear, can cause heart problems and doctors are beginning to recognize the fact that, under emotional stress, especially under the emotion of anger, the blood creates a chemical deposit around the body's ligaments.

Worry, fear, anger, jealousy, and other emotional conditions like these are mental and are the invisible cause of the vast majority of today's most common physical illnesses and problems.

A healthy mind is reflected in a healthy body, and in the same way, an abnormal mental state is expressed as an abnormal physical condition. Thoughts are literally things!

Modern psychology affirms that all the thoughts and emotions that we have thought and felt since we are conscious beings are present in our subconscious mind and are active and subconsciously manifest as tendencies that shape the body in either health or disease and also determine our reactions in life and to different experiences.

This does not mean that a disease is created by a specific thought but is the result of inharmony in mind. Many people die of anguish and emotional pain, outbursts of anger, deep resentment, excessive worry, and other states of mind where there was no specific thought. What you must remember is that the activity of the mind always creates a corresponding physical and an inharmonious mental and emotional state will always create inharmonious conditions in the body and life.

Thoughts are things, they have the power to manifest as physical matter, and they are the cause of all conditions.

Most of us find ourselves immersed in a routine world, a cycle that provides us with security and confidence. The previous planning of tasks indicates the path we should follow. However, when we encounter limitations, we imprison ourselves in thoughts lacking spontaneity and that for the most part, limit our creativity. These, in turn, get worse over time.

Rumination: The Bottleneck in the Cycle of Negativity

Human beings are predisposed to plan and organize our activities. This fills us with security and confidence. However, it limits other fundamental aspects of our life, imaginative capacity and spontaneity are separated.

Thus, we have that, the negative and obsessive thoughts that enter humans involve a series of aspects that decrease the quality of life. One of them is rumination. This phenomenon arises when our thinking remains linked with an element that can be real or imaginary and that as a consequence produces high levels of stress and discomfort.

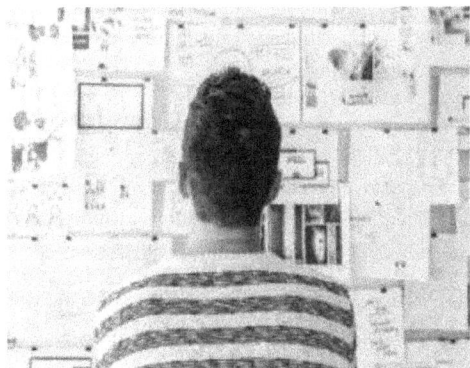

Without realizing it, we start a vicious cycle in which we are called upon by every negative thought or concern, we get used to the feeling of discomfort, and it increases over time.

In this way, we lose our ability to concentrate, and it is more difficult for us to deal with positive thoughts since we usually link all our ideas to those specific situations that we know that will cause us negative feelings. This continuous loop does not allow us to free ourselves from accumulated stress.

This account presents the relationships between the cognitive processes of negative orientation to the problem, concern and rumination, with anxious, depressive symptoms and the present one in difficulties in eating behavior.

Negative problem orientation and trait worry are transdiagnostic factors for panic symptoms and agoraphobia, generalized anxiety disorder, social phobia and behavioral eating, whereas brooding is a transdiagnostic factor for depression, posttraumatic stress disorder and behavioral eating. Reflection has a relationship with social phobia. Results are discussed based on the theoretical model of social phobia and posttraumatic stress.

Repetitive negative thoughts are considered as factors of cognitive vulnerability for various anxiety, mood, and behavior disorders. Those involve an attentive, persistent, frequent cognitive activity, and relatively uncontrollable that focus on the aspects of negatives of the self and the world.

Rumination, in particular, predicts the onset of depression and plays a relevant role both in its maintenance and in its recurrence.

Rumination is defined as a pattern of repetitive thoughts and behaviors that focus attention on oneself, on symptoms, depressive outlets and their causes, meanings and consequences of these symptoms, instead of focusing actively on a solution to solve the circumstances surrounding these symptoms.

Most investigations consider rumination as a two-dimensional construct constituted by two factors: reflection, which is defined as a reflective process whose purpose is to participate in the cognitive problem solving to alleviate the state of low mood; and the reproaches, which consist of rumination negativist or self-reproachful and situations by passively comparing the situation currently with some standard not reached.

In addition to rumination, another of the negative repetitive thoughts is the so-called worry, which is defined as a chain of thought or language activity verbal and images (although rather the first ones) loaded with negative affect and relatively uncontrollable. The worrying process represents an attempted mental problem solving on a subject whose outcome is uncertain. However, it entails the possibility of one or more negative consequences.

Therefore, the concern is closely related to the fear process. Like rumination, worry is a central characteristic of generalized anxiety disorder. However, it is also common in other anxiety disorders and mood.

A cognitive process related to both worry as with rumination is the negative orientation to the problem which is defined as "a system of beliefs that reflect the perception of a problem as a threat to well-being, experiencing doubts about the ability to solve problems, and the tendency to be pessimistic about its result". In a sample of adults, such as negative orientation, the problem turns out to be a predictor of depression.

If gender is considered, women are two times more likely than men to have a depressive disorder; differences that are clear in adolescence and adulthood, although in older people, no differences were found in depression due to gender.

On the other hand, higher prevalence of depression in women has been applied taking into account several theories, among which is the theory of response styles, which suggests that women have a greater ruminative style than men which makes them more vulnerable to depression. In this sense, the reproaches are higher in women, who also have higher scores in depression, negative orientation toward problems and reproaches.

Obsessive thoughts: the Dangers of Rumination

It is natural to stop and reflect on painful experiences or daily worries. With this, we hope to reach a new understanding that reduces our need and allows us to move forward. But this natural process of self-reflection often goes awry. Instead of getting an emotional release, we simply play the same distressing scenes in our head over and over again, feeling even sadder, angry, or agitated.

We relive the scenes of a painful breakup and re-analyze all the nuances of that last conversation. We review in our minds every detail of the last moments before we were affected by a trauma or loss. We relive all the meetings in which our boss criticized us in front of our colleagues, or we rehearsed various versions of a confrontation or discussion that did not end as we would have liked.

This need to ruminate on our worries can occur at any time and occupy our thoughts when we go shopping, when we are in the shower, when we are making dinner, or when we are trying to do our work. Before we know it, our state of mind is already in shambles, and emotions are feeling rawer than ever.

The Hidden Dangers of Getting Caught in a Ruminative Cycle

Rumination is considered a maladaptive form of self-reflection, as it offers some new insights and only intensifies the emotional and psychological distress we already feel. It may seem obvious that such ruminative cycles are emotionally distressing, but less obvious are the significant risks they pose to our mental and physical health.

- Ruminations create a vicious circle that can easily trap us. This urge can be truly addictive, so the more we ruminate, the more we feel compelled to keep doing it.
- Rumination can increase our probability of falling into depression and can prolong the duration of previous depressive episodes.
- It is associated with an increased risk of alcohol abuse. We often drink when we are on the brink of irritability and sadness that stem from our constant musings.
- The phenomenon is associated with an increased risk of eating disorders. Many of us use food to manage the distressing feelings that our own reflections provoke.
- It encourages negative thoughts. Spending such a disproportionate amount of time on negative and painful events can color our general perceptions in such a way that we begin to view other aspects of our lives negatively as well.
- Furthermore, it encourages the procrastination of problems. As an example, often women with ruminative tendencies who find a lump in their breast wait two months longer than women without this tendency to schedule a medical exam. A study confirms that.
- Ruminating thoughts increases our responses to psychological and physiological stress in such a way that the risks of possible cardiovascular disease multiply.

The simple and mere act of thinking corresponds to the intellectual exercise of projecting and enunciating images and ideas in the human mind. Depending on the favorable, pleasant or not approach of them, the thoughts are classified as positive or negative, with the consequent impact on the day-to-day of each one as an individual, and as a society.

Historically, the existence of both lines of thought has always been considered, and an endless number of philosophical, religious and psychological currents have addressed their study and repercussions both individually and collectively.

But it has been in recent years when there has really been a growing interest in these issues, which motivated their greater dissemination both scientific and media, intending to transmit a broader knowledge, which provides more clarity and depth to the influence that they can have the different types of thoughts in the health of the human being, and the development of the interpersonal bonds.

Negative thoughts are those that induce fear, anxiety and stress. Therefore, they can cause us great psychological discomfort, significantly affecting our mental health.

Since we can remember, the head begins to invade us with all kinds of ideas and thoughts. This is more than positive as it helps us develop the cognitive and creative part of our brain. However, what happens in there can also come back against us without warning and with the sole objective of playing all kinds of tricks on us since different types of negative thoughts can appear.

The Most Common Negative Thoughts

Next, I present a list with some of the most common negative thoughts, explaining what each one of them consists of.

Negative thoughts or unreasonable evaluations have often crossed our lives since we are constantly evaluating the situations that are going to present us, but what we have to know is to value ourselves reasonably so that they do not affect us more than necessary and be aware that its content is neither objective. Therefore, I am going to know which are the most common negative thoughts that have surely crossed your mind at some point in your life:

1. Dichotomous thinking

Dichotomous thinking is a rigid and inflexible type of thinking, with no nuances between black and white. Therefore, it is based on the assumption of two mutually exclusive categories, ignoring the intermediate elements and other nuances.

That is, it is about those thoughts that are located in the extremes. For example:

- "You are with me or against me."
- "Either I do it well, or I don't."
- *"All or nothing."*
- *"Now or never."*

2. Fear of what they will say

Who has not ever gone down the street thinking about "what will they say"? This increases especially when we think that we are not dressed properly, or we have to speak in public. Which is very negative for us, since we cannot live pending on others.

Remember that everyone can make mistakes and that what is really important is what you believe about yourself. Sometimes we worry excessively about what others think of us, and in reality, it is impossible to know what others think about you, only that you think you know what they have in their heads. This would be a cognitive distortion, specifically called thought reading.

For example: "If I talk to these people I will speak nothing but nonsense, I will make a fool of myself, and they will reject me."

3. Wanting to have everything under control

When we vehemently believe that something can go wrong, our mind will support this idea and recommend that we abandon our endeavor, with thoughts such as:

- "It sure is going to go wrong."
- "I'm not good at this."

- "It's not worth trying."

There are many negative thoughts that the only thing they will do is that we always stay in the comfort zone. But remember that he who *"does not risk, does not win."* Negative thoughts can cause us to never get out of comfort.

4. Generalize the negative

Some people tend to stick with the negative. For this reason, it is normal that when something bad happens, they believe that it will become a universal norm. Success often comes after a multitude of failures. Saying that something bad will always happen because it happened only once is meaningless.

Falling into the generalization of events is one of the most frequent errors that we can have. You have to be more optimistic about life, and if something bad happens to you today, tomorrow will be another day, but the same thing will not happen to you every day.

We anticipate negative consequences and that predisposition makes us end up confirming what we feared. For example:

- **Anticipatory thinking:** "If I speak in public, I will stutter."

- **Act with the presence of premonitory thought and anxiety:** "I begin to speak and, indeed, as I feared, I am stuttering."

- **Finally, my cognitive evaluation or conclusion would be:** "As I was afraid I have stuttered. *It is best not to speak in public again" (avoidance).*

5. Disqualify both ourselves and the rest

When we enter into conflict with ourselves or with anyone close to us, it is normal for irrational thoughts to arise in our mind, such as:

1. *"This person is worthless."*

2. *"But what nonsense are you saying."*

3. *"I really like you."*

But you should never get carried away by anger or impulsiveness, as it only serves to draw hasty conclusions that, later, we may regret.

6. Dramatize the situation

Who has not ever thought *"what will become of me"* or *"I will never find someone like me again"* after suffering a love breakup? If we want to overcome these situations, it is best not to exaggerate everything and to have future prospects. Lots of people have gone through your thing (or even worse), and all have been able to rebuild their lives and move on. Negative thoughts feed off how dramatic you can be.

Faced with everyday events or symptoms that are actually harmless, we experience terrible consequences, generating great fears that, if not treated properly, will condition our lives.

It is very good to think that we can do everything and that we are capable of reaching the end of the world. Still, one thing must be clear, and that is that many times this can become a problem for ourselves because by failing to meet these expectations, we can generate large doses of sadness or anxiety.

Learn from Example

Jim has social anxiety problems. He usually locks himself at home and hardly ever goes out due to his anxiety, although he would like to be able to do so and meet people.

A good friend invited him out for dinner on a Saturday with a group of people, most of them unknown to Jim. It is a very difficult situation for him, normally he would reject the proposal, but this time he decided to pose it as a personal challenge and go. He immediately experienced anxiety and negative thoughts, along with the desire not to go. However, he plucked up his courage and went before, and during dinner, he tried to "answer" his negative thoughts and think rationally.

His thoughts were:

- **Negative thought:** *I will be rejected. They'll think I'm weird. It is best to stay at home/arbitrary inference.*
- **Negative thought**: *I'm useless, I don't know how to be with people/classification*
- **Negative thinking**: *Everyone will be looking at me, thinking badly of me/mind-reading*
- **Negative thinking:** *Nobody likes me /overgeneralization*

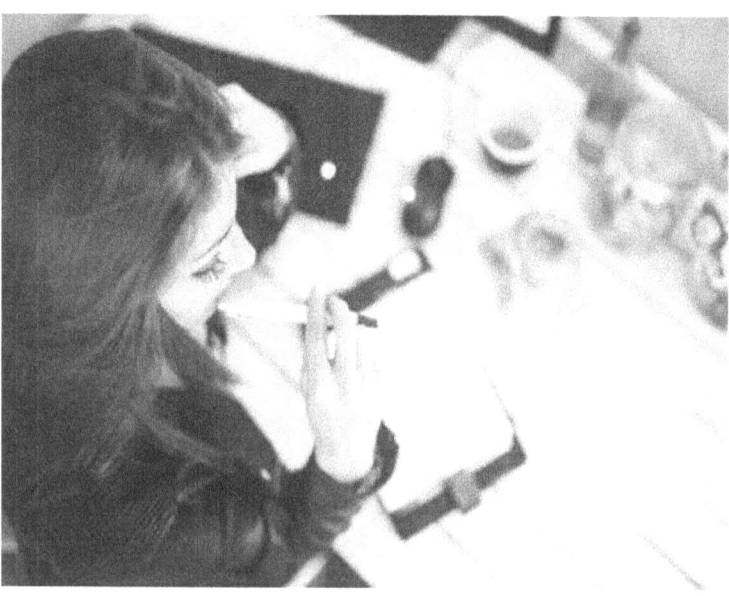

I Am Sorry But, Negative Thoughts Don't Go Away

Being aware of negative thoughts and analyzing them rationally is the first step. We can give them the weight they deserve, but it won't make the thoughts go away! Nor will it succeed in forcing us to "think positive".

- Jim will continue to feel insecure in social situations, and although he realizes that his thoughts are irrational, it is normal that he continues to have that feeling.

It happens to all of us, or has it ever happened to us: knowing that a negative thought is irrational or exaggerated. But even so, we cannot get rid of it.

Even on many occasions, that negative thought, despite being exaggerated or making me suffer a lot, maybe partly right.

I give you an example:

- Imagine that I have had a headache for days, and in my mind, I begin to elaborate the thought that it could be something serious, I can even start looking on the Internet... and convince myself that it is most likely a brain tumor. It generates terrible anguish and a mental movie in which I die unexpectedly in a few months.

If I "try not to think" about that negative film, I probably will not succeed, the usual thing is that it distracts me for a while and the worry comes back (maybe even more strongly). It is also probable that rationally I see that I'm exaggerating: but I'm not capable of stopping worrying.

If we analyze this negative thought: "I'm sure it's a brain tumor, I'm going to die" we see that it is irrational because it is exaggerated and because it takes the worst of the options for granted ... but we can't really say that it's not true: because I don't know. Maybe yes, maybe it's a brain tumor.

The issue is that it can be something very serious or not; that concern is only one of the possibilities. It could be a tumor, or it could be a tension headache, I don't know.

If I say to myself "I'm an exaggeration, it sure is nothing!" That's also just one of the options, so a part of me keeps thinking. "Okay, it might be nothing, but what if it is?" And I get hooked again. Back to square one.

Thought Influences Action: Negativity Calls for More Negativity

If we really think that something can go wrong, it is obvious that it will go wrong. This is called a self-fulfilling prophecy. But what happened will not be a matter of fate or bad luck as some say, but of the negativity that invades our mind and affects our capacity for action. It will produce a chain effect with dire consequences for our self-esteem.

According to Beck (1983), negative thoughts are rigid, inflexible, absolutist. They also have the form of *"I have to"*, *"I must think of"*. On the other hand, positive thoughts are flexible, possible, and adaptive. And they have the form of *"I would like it to"*, *"I would like it to."*

Every day, our brain keeps all the information experienced throughout the day and saves it from processing it in the memory drawer. A day we have 50,000 thoughts of which 10,000 are negative, and there are also times that certain thoughts can lead us to fall into the confusion of whether they are good or bad for us and if we do not know how to question them they can do us a lot of harm.

When we start to have negative thoughts about the same topic, these can end up really hurting us, since they get bigger and bigger at the same time that we believe them more strongly.

All negative thoughts do is take away our energy and take away all the strength and vitality that we have from the moment we get up until we get into bed.

The more I believe my negative thoughts, they become stronger, taking root in our thinking style, and it is much more difficult to avoid them.

Sometimes negative thoughts can hurt, so much so that they can condition your life and your character. Since in the end these thoughts, if we do not know how to question them, can damage our way of valuing ourselves (self-esteem) or make us believe that harmless situations or symptoms are a potential danger.

Why do we feed negative thinking if it really hurts us?

It can be said that the initial problem of this is when the first bad thoughts assail us, that if we do not know how to deal with them, they end up haunting our minds more.

The typical phrase of "don't think about it anymore and forget it" is a mistake since the more we think about forgetting that thought that is hurting us, the more present we have it, in such a way that the idea ends up haunting us almost in a cyclical way and continues in our head and can become an obsession.

In our day-to-day life, the brain automatically interprets everything that surrounds us and, although in most cases, the messages it offers us are positive and useful, it can also confuse us. Psychologists have studied in depth what is known as "automatic negative thoughts" (known in the world as ANT, for its acronym in English – *automatic negative thoughts*): pernicious ideas that appear in our head without us looking for them and constitute a dangerous source of disturbing emotions.

Although ANTs have been the subject of study by many psychologists and psychiatrists, it was one of the founders of cognitive therapies, the American doctor Aaron Temkin Beck. The latter most contributed to its definition in the 1960s. Beck believed that ANTs were determinant in our well-being, or rather in our discomfort.

In his opinion, these negative thoughts sabotage the best of ourselves and, if we do not know how to control ourselves, they end up creating a situation of insecurity, anxiety and anger that, in turn, generates new ANTs. A vicious cycle from which it is not easy to get out, in which negative thoughts are repeated.

These negative thoughts sabotage the best of ourselves and, if we do not know how to control ourselves, they end up creating a situation of infidelity and anger.

Luckily, there are techniques to escape this dangerous brain network. Neural plasticity, which we know better and better, shows that the brain is fickle: we can all kill ANTs and put positive thoughts in their place. But to do this, the first thing we have to do is identify these and understand that these are thoughts for which we are not responsible (at least not consciously).

Unmasking Our Inner Critic

Behind most feelings of discomfort are one or more ANTs, which are not always easy to notice. To identify them, we must first know what three main characteristics these thoughts fulfill:

- **They are specific messages**

ANTs usually have a specific and recurring form, easily identifiable in our inner speech. Since our evil Jiminy Cricket always speaks in the same way, it is easy to unmask him. In general, these are messages that seem shorthand, composed of a short phrase that appears in our head over and over again, in the form of memories, assumptions or self-reproaches, such as the reconstruction of a past event ("if I had done X, there would be no past X"), the fictitious creation of a future event ("I always do wrong X, and in the future, the same thing will happen again"), or a guilty demand (" I should have done X, I should have done X.").

- **They are credible messages**

ANTs arise automatically, spontaneously: they suddenly enter the mind, without our having made any prior judgment of the situation. But, despite the lack of solidity of their arguments, we perceive them as absolute truths, as ideas that we have been reflecting on for a long time; and that is where their danger lies: we take for granted something that is not.

If we can identify these thoughts, to analyze them cold, we will be able to realize how ridiculous they are most of the time.

Although ANT from the outside may seem ridiculous, the person who suffers them considers them very real and credible, precisely because they do not stop to analyze them (hence the positive thing that is to share these with third parties). We take them for valid, without questioning them, because they are experienced as spontaneous absolute truths, something that can be solved if we learn to analyze them logically to verify that their conclusions are exaggerated.

- **They are thoughtless messages**

To know how to keep these negative thoughts at bay (ending them completely is impossible), we must realize that our inner voice only offers us one point of view: ANTs respond to the automation of the brain, which does not include a prior reflection of the brain. Judgment issued, but that seems most logical. If we can identify these thoughts, to analyze them coldly and with caution, we will be able to realize how ridiculous they are on most occasions, and we will be able to neutralize them.

The Chain of Negative Thoughts

It is important to understand how we find ourselves in the pit of negativity. There is a chain, a stimulus which causes us to react in the said way. Below I have drawn some of the most common examples which can help us understand what goes around negative thinking, in general:

- **"Tomorrow I'm going to fail the meeting"**

What worries me about the meeting? Not having prepared the subject enough. What is the first one that I face in the company? Do I think like this every time I'm under pressure?

Whatever the answer, I will not be able to know what will happen until it happens. To worry is to suffer twice, the first time by assuming that the meeting will go wrong and the second if it happens in the end. But if it goes well? We have wasted that time on unnecessary discomfort.

- **"You sure are thinking I'm a mess"**

As social beings that we are, it is inevitable to take into account the opinion or impression we make on other people but deciding whether or not to do something based on what others will think is a losing battle, no matter what we do. We will not be able to control what they will say.

- **"If I fail this exam I will be unable to move forward"**

Have I failed the rest of the subjects? If the answer is no, visualizing such negative consequences will not help me, quite the opposite.

If I finally fail the exam, I will give credibility to what I thought ("I was right") and it may decrease my motivation to keep trying for the rest of the course. If I finally get worse grades, it won't be because of my divinatory skills, but because I gave up before my time what was in my power to change.

- **"Today, my neighbor has not greeted me. He is rude"**

If every time we come across him, we don't get an answer, it seems reasonable to think about it, but to draw hasty conclusions without sufficient argument. Is he rude, or is he in a hurry? What if you haven't heard us?

- **"What I have achieved has no merit, it has been very easy"**

We are used to valuing as positive those things that go out of our routine (a trip, a surprise) and to normalize the importance of **the small pleasures** of our day to day (a coffee with a friend, a compliment, a smile).

Something similar happens to us with our achievements. If we detract from what we achieve, we are tripping ourselves. We don't have to wait for big events to assess ourselves.

- **"I have to be able to do it"**

Phrases that begin with I have to or must do not usually have a good prognosis. When we use these types of messages, we are adding extra pressure to what we want to do, feeling bad if we do not comply. The connotation of requirement decreases if we replace it with "I would like".

These approaches are just brushstrokes of the wide range of nuances and variables that exist in each situation that each of us experiences, which is why it is so important to contextualize what happens to us to avoid damaging ourselves with what we think.

Chapter II: Negativity and Us

The pathologies related to anxiety and depression almost always involve a significant degree of catastrophic thinking. In other words, patients tend to think, imagine, and believe in the worst outcomes for their problems and doubts, often fantasizing about tragic scenarios of events that hardly ever happen to them or most people.

Let's start with some examples that capture this feature well:

- A person with panic disorder often thinks that their pounding heartbeat will lead to a heart attack or that their headaches are the beginning of a stroke.
- A man with generalized anxiety disorder talks on the phone with his wife, who tells him that he is about to take a bus with the children; the man thinks that one of the children may fall under the bus's wheels and die.
- A person with depression believes that his family does not love him, imagines that in a few years, he will end up abandoned, alone, and die ill in a public asylum for homeless people.

The above are just some examples representing the typical case of catastrophism, not only because of the tragic scenario that the patient has in his consciousness, but also very important because the feared event has never happened to him and because the chances of it happening are very small. However, the person cannot stop thinking about it, with the consequent suffering that this causes.

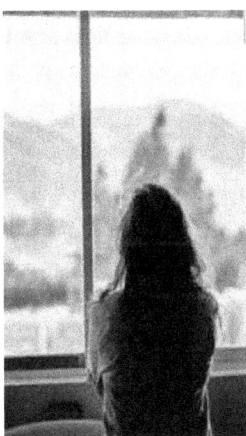

Let's simply say that a person thinks, believes, and fears an infinite number of times a negative event that does not happen. Countless times they are is wrong, but for some reason, they fail to incorporate the simple evidence that what they fear does not happen. Therefore, they continue with heeding tragic thoughts in their head.

It is as if we wake up every day thinking and believing that when we look out the window, we will see a beautiful landscape of sea and mountains, but instead, we find a gloomy building lung.

And even though today and all the previous mornings, I have seen the same building lung, it does not matter. I wake up tomorrow with the belief that the beautiful landscape will appear before me. Absurd, right?

Well, this is how absurd it should sound to us that every day we experience fear of negative events that have never happened. But of course, it is simpler to notice the folly with a positive fact than with a negative one, something that is related to the nature and origin of catastrophic thinking.

In the first instance, millions of years of evolution have left indelible marks on the human brain, among which is an increased facility to react with fear of ambiguity and uncertainty. Let's think of an organism living in a primitive environment, in a natural environment such as a forest or jungle. You hear an atypical sound among the trees.

Reacting with a defensive response such as fear would facilitate their survival in the face of a predator's possible presence. I have stated this example before too. Conversely, an "upbeat" reaction such as continuing without alerting yourself could lead to death.

In the archaic environment that has been present during the millions of years of evolution of life. Fear turns out to be a critical adaptation without which it cannot survive, so today, we show this increased facility to react defensively to the uncertain. Now, it happens that the fear reaction involves several levels and response systems, among which is the cognitive one. That is the origin of catastrophism.

It is the cognitive expression of an evolutionarily facilitated tendency. In this way, thinking about the worst possible outcomes facilitates adaptation to an objectively more hostile environment, where dangers were more frequent than in our modern environments.

On the contrary, being positive and optimistic carried the risk of not reacting promptly to a threat that, if real, would leave us out of the evolutionary chain. All of this has changed in the modern and civilized environments in which most of today's humans move, yet primitive reactions continue in our deep brain, relics of our primitive past.

Now, the previous thesis partially explains the problem of catastrophism as a cognitive style. While it is true that it gives us a solid clue to understanding why we react easily with fear and catastrophic thinking to ambiguous situations and why being optimistic is not intuitive and natural for us?

On the other hand, it leaves open the question about why some people seem to become entrenched in catastrophic thinking that leads to fear, suffering even the development of psychological disorders while others succeed in taming the primitive being that is inside us.

In other words, why in catastrophic thinking, does it become frequent, intense, and long-lasting in some, while it is sporadic, mild, and fleeting in others? As is often the case, there is no single answer to this question.

Neuroscientific research has documented that there are individual differences due to hereditary factors. After all, all the organs of the body carry their genetic factory stamp. The brain does not have to be an exception. While this is very interesting, it exceeds the objectives of this chapter.

Second, reacting with fear involves learning. Although, as an emotional pattern, the fear response is innate, what we learn is what to react to. Early experiences of intense stress predispose to the lability of the emotional system. Thus, living strongly stressful childhood experiences, living in an emotionally unstable climate during the first years leaves the system more predisposed to shoot, with more intensity and frequency.

Somehow, the first years leave an imprint, if during them we have gone through stressful experiences, we are left with the general message that "our environment is dangerous, hostile and therefore, we must always be prepared to defend ourselves," and from there we derive a facility from thinking catastrophically, because somehow in the first years we have verified that "it is better to always be prepared."

Another critical factor in maintaining catastrophic thinking relates to what we do when such thoughts appear. That is, once the tragic thoughts have appeared in our minds, and we feel anxious, what do we do? What do we say to ourselves? How do we deal with them? This topic has special relevance to the psychological clinic as it is one of the edges through which we can operate to reduce the phenomenon.

In some cases, the person who has a catastrophic thought not only reacts emotionally with anxiety, as an involuntary process but also says or performs behaviors aimed at reducing that anxiety without questioning the integrity of the catastrophic thought. Somehow, they act under the influence that what they think is true, simply because they think it as if cognitions had their weight like that of facts. This is a mistake.

Having a mental image frequently in my consciousness does not make the fact described by that image objectively more probable. One of the most characteristic examples is found in patients who suffer from health anxiety, who, with minimal abdominal discomfort, believe they have a malignant tumor.

Thinking about the tumor, imagining the diagnosis and treatment of a disease such as cancer does not increase the probability of suffering. Generally, under the influence of an irrationally triggered fear, these patients repeatedly go to the doctor for reassurance in the complete absence of evidence. Which they easily achieve because they only suffer from simple indigestion, information that they already had as they had been through this situation many times.

In this way, unnecessary visits to the doctor turn into reinsurance behaviors that prevent a simple verification process that, in the long run, would lead to the extinction of fear. What was thought simply does not happen. The problem is compounded by the fact that while ideas are not true, it does happen that the frequency with which we think about them makes them seem subjectively more likely, a phenomenon known as subjective probability or heuristic probability.

Our brain subjectively estimates the probability of an event according to two types of analysis. One follows logical and rational guidelines, such as those derived from a statistic that the airplane is the safest means of transport of all.

However, there is also an estimate of the probability based on the times we have thought about a certain fact. The more we think about it, the more likely we feel it, regardless of the objective knowledge. For this reason, those who suffer from a flying phobia feel that the plane will crash because they have simply thought about it countless times.

This also explains why the person in our previous example, who suffered from health anxiety, feels that he or she is very likely to develop cancer, nothing more, and nothing less than because she frequently thinks about it.

This is what we call heuristic or subjective probability, a process that we could summarize by saying that on some occasions when we frequently think about something, we end up not distinguishing how much of it is objectively true and how much we have invented it.

In some people, the factors above converge more than in others in the same direction, resulting in the fear reaction and its cognitive counterpart, catastrophic thinking, being expressed with more frequency, intensity, and duration.

If we all share a biologically and evolutionarily facilitated tendency to react with anxiety, there are individual differences in what we have inherited, in what we learned during the critical years of childhood, and in how we deal with catastrophic cognitions once presented.

Why Do We Sigh? How Does It Relate to Stress?

This act sometimes has something romantic about it, as if in that exhalation, we let go of our sadness, the regret of longing, or the longing to be in love. For many, sighing is one more language of love and is often even poetically defined as the soul's complaint. However, is there any reality in all this?

The truth is that very little. Despite this, there is one aspect that we must be very clear about: sighing is a decisive physiological process. Doing so is decisive for lung health, and for the emotional aspect. What's more, the brain needs it to the point that many neurologists define this mechanism as the "mental reset" button.

Let's learn more about it below.

"Our crying is such a small thing; Sighs are such a small thing… However, for such small things, you and we will die". – Emily Dickinson

Why do we sigh?

Take a moment to answer these questions: How many times a day do you sigh? Are you one of those who sigh every two by three? Beyond looking like the classic questions that every child would ask, it should be noted that something as every day as sighing is key to many living beings' integral health.

Because not only do people do it, but if we look closely at our pets, we will see how our dogs or cats do it. Is it that they too fall in love, are they sad or frustrated? We do not know, but what we do know is that this mechanism is very important to preserve lung health.

Furthermore, if we do not carry out these periodic inhalations throughout the day, we will die.

The sighs, a vital reflection

Sigh to live. It seems like a phrase taken from a commercial, but it is not. Now we understand this mechanism much more, to the point that a work published in the journal nature defines it as a vital reflection. We have discovered that we have two small groups of nerve cells in the brain stem that orchestrate this process.

This set of cells' main task is to automatically take care of breathing, sleep, and heart rate. Now we know that it also activates the sigh mechanism.

And for what purpose? If we ask ourselves why we sigh, the answer is simple: prevent the alveoli from collapsing. There are times when these small sacs that form the lungs and that control the exchange between oxygen and carbon dioxide get stuck.

What the sigh does is inflate the collapsed alveoli with more air than normal to reactivate its function.

If we did not, we would start to suffer from lung failure.

The author of this research, Dr. Jack Feldman, professor of neurobiology at the University of Los Angeles School of Medicine, tells us something just as interesting. The brain activates different breaths thanks to neuropeptides, which mediate normal breaths, yawning, coughing, laughing, and crying.

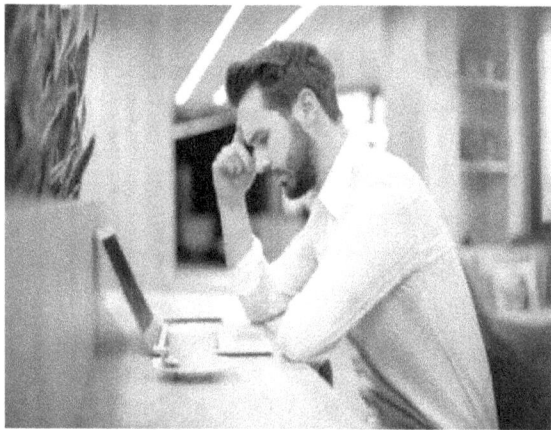

Sighs are also regulated by just over 200 neurons—a very small group of nerve cells capable of fulfilling our survival's vital mission.

When you're stressed, do you sigh more?

Sighs seemed to us until not long ago, with simple long and deep breaths associated with **sadness** and emotional discomfort. Well, now we know that its role is to fill the alveoli with air. However, is that your only function? The truth is that they fulfill more tasks for us.

- **Sighs increase in frequency when we suffer from stress and even certain psychiatric conditions**: **bipolar disorder**, schizophrenia, psychosis. Any state in which our emotional state is of great intensity, sighs will appear. They do it to release tension and let go of the anxiety that the mind and body are subjected to.

- On the other hand, **studies such** as those carried out at the University of Leuven, in Belgium, show us something else. **To the question of why we sigh, we must add another answer: to restore balance in the brain**. It is like resetting the mind, like bringing oxygen inside to hide negativity.

This explains why we can't help but breathe long sighs when gripped by frustration, **disappointment**, sadness, nostalgia, and even boredom. **A sigh not only stretches the pulmonary alveoli, filling them with air. By doing so, a feeling of mental relief is also generated**, we oxygenate ourselves, we obtain calm, and our whole organism recovers its precious homeostasis.

How Do Negativity and Constant Complaining Affect our Brains?

One friend meets another. In five minutes, the first one is overwhelmed and speechless when listening to his interlocutor's complaints. Complaints related to his parents, his brother, the lack of employment, the absence of a partner, the terrible health service, the lack of awareness of his neighbors, and the government's arbitrary measures.

There are situations in life that undoubtedly merit complaining, as a natural reaction to release tensions accumulated by the event itself. The loss of a close family member, being unemployed due to a staff cut, a divorce, or a serious illness are painful experiences for which a complaint can awaken our empathy.

"He had been a man who reveled in how awful his life was and would rather complain than change it." – John Katzenbach

However, some people make complaints about their daily bread. Furthermore, they think that all the "good people" in the world are obliged to listen to those lamentations repeatedly because otherwise, they would prove that they are insensitive or selfish.

Contemporary complaints

Living in the current age is not easy. We are constantly bombarded by news, mostly painful or worrying. Additionally, we must tolerate grumpy bosses or bounced colleagues, not counting the personal problems we are exposed to, such as losses, illnesses, and a bag full of situations that at times become suffocating.

Faced with such a scenario, we generally have two options: Analyze each situation, look for the most appropriate way out, or resist and adopt the complaint's position. The worrying thing about this second option is that it becomes a habit that limits our potential and generates a negative attitude in those around us.

We could think that complaining is a kind of catharsis in the face of pressure, and it may, at times, fulfill this function. However, without our noticing it, the complaint can become a habit that we repeat like a vicious circle and that over time will become the automatic response to difficulties.

Consequences in our brain

According to research carried out by various neuroscientists, the frequency and emotional intensity with which we will depend on whether our brain undergoes significant changes. This is because during this condition of constant frustration and impotence, the brain releases hormones such as norepinephrine, cortisol, and adrenaline that end up altering the normal functioning of this organ.

Some scientists even claim that being repeatedly exposed to the complaint deteriorates or eliminates the neural connections present in our brain's hippocampus. That is precisely the area in charge of finding solutions to the problems that afflict us.

The insistence on the complaint is a way of negatively conditioning ourselves, which generates rejection in others and ends up deteriorating our family, couple, or work relationships. It is a condition of dependence and, therefore, of immaturity and passivity in the face of problems.

Negative Thinking and Cognitive Decline: the Wear and Tear of Our Brain

Negative thinking and cognitive decline are closely related. A factor that would increase, according to several studies, the risk of suffering memory loss, language, attention, or orientation problems in advanced ages, would be to fall into those mental patterns in which negativity is constant and chronic. We are facing the fact that we should consider and bear in mind.

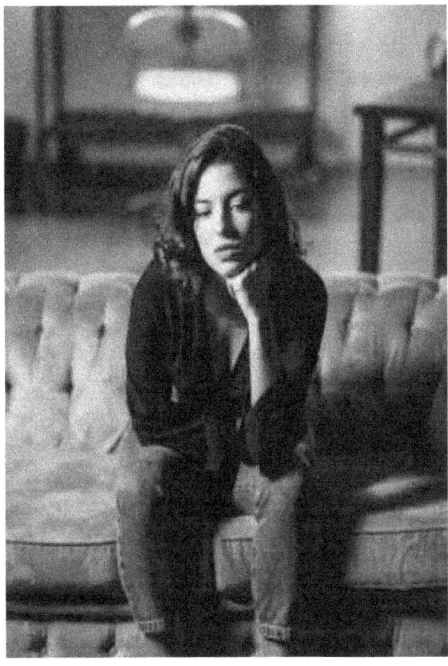

We know it, most of us are clear that what we think favors or limits our quality of life. What's more, it is not just every interpretation we make of what surrounds us or what happens to optimize our well-being or intensify suffering. It is also our feelings and those emotional states that affect, in turn, many of the neurological processes.

We cannot forget, for example, the effect that chronic stress has on areas such as the hippocampus, that region related to memory. In psychological states in which worry is constant and negativity or anguish, the formation of new neurons is seriously limited. With which, over the years, it will not only be increasingly difficult for us to take on new learning; also, the connection between nerve cells loses quality.

Negative thinking and cognitive decline, how are they related?

We all go through times when worry accompanies us like a storm cloud in summer. It's intense, but it doesn't last long. Soon, things change, we find strategies to solve these problems, and we regain stability and calm. Experiencing these situations is completely normal, and none of them affects a neurological level.

What's more, the simple fact of trying to find answers, to be creative, and apply resources to face difficulties, reverts to brain health: we gain flexibility and cognitive reserve. Now, the problem comes when that time of worry becomes chronic. Our mental focus falls into the whirlwind of chronic negativity, seeing no light at the end of the tunnel or the sky through a window.

If this approach is constant throughout a good part of our lives, the risk of suffering cognitive deficits increases. What's more, this fact, added to other factors, increases the probability of Alzheimer's suffering.

The Cognitive Debt Hypothesis

Robert Howard is a Professor of Psychiatry at University College London. In 2015, because of a study, he proposed an already recognized and accepted concept called the cognitive debt hypothesis. According to this idea, repetitive and chronic negative thinking creates damage to the brain and hence cognitive failures (debts) when reaching certain ages.

Another experimental work was carried out to validate this idea, which has seen the light very a few weeks ago. Dr. Natalie Marchant from this same university followed 292 elderly people over five years to demonstrate this hypothesis.

The data appears in the journal Alzheimer's & Dementia. They are as follows:

- **Negative thinking and cognitive decline are related. People with a ruminant, obsessive, and adverse thought pattern end up showing problems in attention, memory, language, and spatial orientation.**

- **Likewise, another no less serious factor appears: Magnetic resonances showed an increase in the deposits of beta-amyloid and tau proteins, which form the classic plaques in neurons, preventing communication between them. This is evidence of the Alzheimer's marker.**

The relationship of anxiety and depression in later life

We know that negative thinking and cognitive decline are closely related. However, there is a trigger behind it. This reasoning pattern devoid of optimism, flexibility, hope, and creativity results from conditions such as anxiety or depression.

This is what Dr. Amy Gimson points out through research carried out at the University of Southampton, United Kingdom.

Mood disorders and loneliness

According to this proposal, it is very common for many people between 55 and 60 to suffer from these mood disorders, often associated with work, family, personal and existential crises. What's more, another factor that we see too often is loneliness.

We are shaping a much more connected, yet lonelier society. We lack quality links. We lack mechanisms to integrate people of any age into daily life so that they interact, set goals on the horizon, continue creating links and nurturing hopes and illusions for the future.

All of these ingredients act as resistance mechanisms for dementias and cognitive deficits. This alone does not prevent Alzheimer's development, but, perhaps, we delay its appearance and gain time and quality of life.

The vicious circle of anger: when emotions get you trapped

The vicious cycle of anger is the basis of many self-destructive behaviors that break relationships and cause uncomfortable situations that fuel regret sooner or later. The impact of this psychological dimension is usually immense if we do not manage it properly. What happens is that not all of us are qualified in this essential life competence.

Dante placed the sins committed by anger in the seventh circle. In turn, he divided it into three more, somewhat smaller and made of stone because, according to him, this aspect of the human being leads us to commit multiple acts, such as an insult or different forms of violence. This area of hell was guarded in turn by a mythological and imposing figure: the minotaur.

Few emotions have more negative and adverse connotations than anger. However, it is important to know that it fulfills its function from a psychological point of view. It is indispensable in our emotional and behavioral repertoire because anger makes us react to injustices, to what hurts us, or challenges our values.

We all have the full right to experience anger, but we also must know how to handle it. If we do it intelligently, we will generate adequate changes to regain balance and feel better.

We could safely say that anger has many similarities to fear. On a psychological level, both emotions make us run away from something or fight against that something. There is no middle ground. The mind and the organism are in survival mode because there is something that bothers us, that hurts us, and that threatens our integrity in some way and, as such, we feel the need to escape or act.

However, few people understand this emotion. We tend to label anger negatively without knowing that it holds great transformative power. It propels us to action and, in general, acting is often an opportunity to change.

Well-directed anger can allow us to solve complex problems and situations. However, before doing so, we need to understand their anatomy and the vicious cycle of anger.

Why do we feel anger?

Anger is a state that can range from simple annoyance to rage. It can be caused by disappointment, frustration, receiving an insult, and injustice, which violates our values and physical integrity. Likewise, this emotion goes through an intense physical activation very similar to that of fear: the heart races, the muscles tense, and what is more worrying, the brain stops thinking in a rational way to allow itself to be hijacked by emotions.

Now there is an important fact about anger that we must know. This emotion can gain intensity if we "feed" it is far from managing it. We let it gain in intensity. And in what way do we nurture or make this emotion bigger? Through the vicious cycle of anger.

The vicious circle of anger, what is it?

The vicious cycle of anger is a trap that we create and strengthen through our thoughts. Studies such as those carried out by the Texas Department of Psychobiology affect the fact that this mechanism occurs when anger is very intense.

It is at that moment that said emotion acts as a cognitive numbing. We put aside our capacity for reflection, and a series of very problematic processes ignite. *They are as follows:*

- On the one hand, the triggering factor causes us annoyance, anger, or rage.

- Physiological dimensions. Psychophysiological activation is very intense. It stresses us, blocks us, and places us in a very complex state where we can end up hitting, screaming, or even breaking down in tears.

- The accumulated emotions. Despite our physiological reactions, anger tends to build up; it integrates within us, altering our balance, distorting everything.

- Altered thoughts. When we swallow our emotions and do not manage them, thinking is altered and changes. That's when everything bothers us. When we start to lose patience, distrust, frustration, and exhaustion arise.

- Distorted reality. When thought is suspended in negativity, pent-up anger, and discomfort, the external world changes, everything turns gray, nothing attracts us, at the least we jump for nothing, and almost anything makes us angry. Almost without realizing it, we experience anger and rage over anything.

People Addicted to Negativity: Six Characteristics

We all know someone prone to see things through a pessimistic perspective. We don't know why, but each time we're with that guy, we see how our mood gets worse, and our urge to escape increases by the minute. This is because we met one of those people who are addicted to negativity.

They seem not much of the time to know their disservice to the people around them. Their pessimism is infectious, which encourages others to turn away from them in the long run. They are usually not evil people, but they are very difficult in their way of seeing things. No one enjoys being reminded of the world's negative stuff.

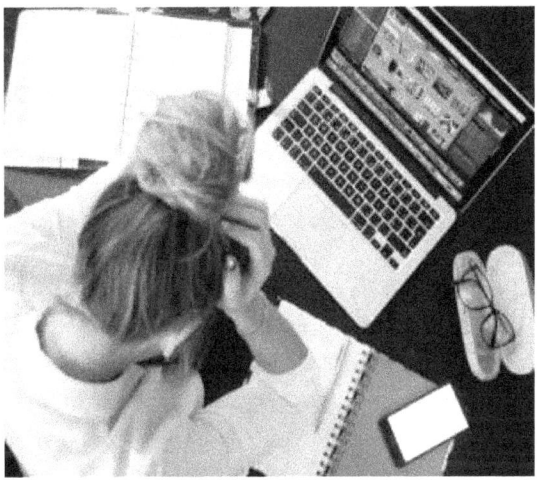

Individuals addicted to negativity cannot see the light in the clouds of hurricanes or note the only cloud in a sky dominated by a burning sun.

If they don't do their part to alter their outlook, we can do nothing for them. So, if we want to support them, the first thing we need to do is to inspire them to make a move, to make the decision.

Six characteristics of people addicted to negativity

1. **They worry about trivial issues**

People addicted to negativity drown in a glass of water. For them, the shattering of a plate is a world drama that they can swap for a new one in a few hours. They become cynical thinking about the future instead of enjoying the day to day, making them even more pessimistic.

They don't know how to assign proper importance to each item, and their propensity to exaggerate something will lead them to be accused of being unreliable. We all recall the story of Peter and the Wolf and its tragic end.

2. **They ignore the positive**

It does not matter if they had a great day at work if they had a gift or received good news. They only focus on those parts of their life that they don't like, completely ignoring the good times.

They are not aware of their life by avoiding the positive, and when they reflect, they appear to come to the logical conclusion of their impression that they are very bad, or that their worth is very poor. They don't care about their happiness. They just stay stuck in the loop of misfortunes that their mind manipulates.

3. **They are unable to accept a compliment**

They respond poorly when someone gives them a compliment or a threat. So much negativity also affects their self-esteem, and any flattering remark would be considered an offense.

They think others are laughing at them when they just want to be nice. They cannot accept that they, too, have values, no matter how hard it is to believe.

4. **They only talk about their problems: there is hardly room in their head for those of others**

They love to show how horrible their life is for them, but they don't care how others feel. They do not know how to listen, and they are egotistical: theirs are always worse. The few occasions they let somebody take part in their monologue are because they have something to object to. Sometimes this lack of empathy leads to confrontations with others, especially when a limit is exceeded.

Of course, they have the need to continually vent, which is quite burdensome.

5. **They take very little risks**

They worry so much about what others think of them. Any negative remark is having an unsettling impact on them. They base their own opinion on others' opinions, lacking in objectivity, which leads them to be very insecure and dependent.

They are so afraid of suffering because of what others might say or do that they do not hesitate to make their own "mental videos" in which they are often abused or harmed (something we all do, but with more "special effects"). They prefer to take a few chances in this way and to defend themselves (they believe that they already take plenty, or that they have "too many open fronts").

6. **They can become very paranoid**

People who are addicted to the negative are highly paranoid. A laugh out of place or a furtive smile makes them think we're talking ill of them. This makes those around them very suspicious of them, strengthening others' urge to get away from them.

Their actions can be hard to bear and even intolerable. You should be careful and try to understand why they're behaving like this.

Much of the time, their actions are the product of a series of unpleasant experiences that have not been treated well. It's never too late to relearn that not everything in life is black or white: we live in grey surroundings. Good days and bad days are going to take place, but not everyone has to be terrible.

The Science of Guilt

Guilt is considered one of the "negative" emotions that we can experience throughout our lives on numerous occasions. Nobody likes to experience this emotion as it makes us feel bad, but it is necessary to correct our environment.

This emotion arises from the belief or feeling of having violated personal or social-ethical norms towards others (for which another person is harmed) or towards oneself. We can find a pang of cause-effect guilt, we did something that we thought we should not have done, or conversely, we did not do something that we believed should have been done, and now we feel bad.

Guilt is a mechanism in which, based on an act or omission, we make a "moral judgment" of our behavior (including our thoughts) and "rule" that we have made a mistake, and we should be punished. Being a judgment that we make of our behaviors (and thoughts), guilt is a very subjective emotion, since it is part of that interpretation that we make of our actions. Hence, sometimes it is so destructive. In most cases, there is no objective fact that initiates the person's sequence to feel guilty for what has happened or has stopped happening.

Main elements of guilt

There are three main elements of which guilt consists:

- The causal act, real or imaginary.
- The negative perception or self-assessment of the act by the person (bad conscience)
- The unpleasant emotion derived from guilt proper (remorse)

The feeling of guilt can easily lead to sadness, shame, anxiety, and self-pity, causing a host of emotions that make us feel bad and feed into each other, making it difficult to identify and therefore overcome.

Guilt can go in two directions:

• **Intrinsic:** It is that discomfort that invades us for having committed an act (or the absence of it) and that we have been harmed for that reason. For example, taking an exam, failing it, and thinking, "If I had studied more..." Feeling guilty for not having studied enough to face the exam and be able to pass it.

• **Extrinsic:** It arises when we carry out a behavior (or the absence of it), and therefore another person (different from ourselves) is harmed. For example, being in the middle of an argument with a friend and you disrespecting him makes your friend feel hurt. You feel guilty for having hurt the person.

How does guilt manifest itself?

Sometimes, the feeling of guilt can become so strong that it can noticeably manifest itself through the following signs:

- **Physical:** The psychophysiological activation of the feeling of guilt manifests with pain in the chest, stomach, pressure in the head, and discomfort in the back.
- **Emotional:** Irritability, nervousness, and, frequently, we identify it as something like sadness.
- **Cognitive:** Self-reproaches, self-accusations, and destructive thoughts of self-esteem and self-worth.

When guilt turns pathological

An emotion becomes pathological when it is experienced habitually, very regularly, frequently becoming a very strong and invasive feeling, so much so that it hinders our day-to-day life. We stop being functional at different levels (work, social, family), and we drift at the mercy of emotion.

Guilt can be pathological by excess, and by default, there is a distortion of awareness of the situation in both cases. The excessive or inappropriate feeling of guilt is closely linked to depression, as a symptom of depressive episodes, where the person tends to constantly self-recriminate. You start to feel guilty about being depressed and not being able to feel the way others do.

Pathological guilt is also present in obsessive-compulsive disorders (characterized by its high demand and perfectionism), in phobias and addictions. In such cases, guilt operates as part of the problem. It is not healthy guilt that leads to repair or redirect behavior. Rather, it works as a factor of constant emotional punishment, which generally aggravates the central problem.

Feelings of guilt and unworthiness are very intense, based on trivial incidents or minor guilt from the past, which now turns into a mountain of unworthiness and damage. For example: "I am a monster," "I am worth nothing," "I am to blame for the death of...". That is, the person feels guilty without having done something objectively wrong or even without knowing why.

This type of guilt, referring to behaviors beyond the control of the person, is destructive and prevents them from experiencing joy for the behaviors they perform correctly. Since these go unnoticed, they lack value and importance, ultimately, enjoy life.

There are many types of negative thoughts that can harm you. These are generally automatic ideas, some of which are nothing more than introjected beliefs; that is, beliefs that your parents or other significant adults transmitted to you during your first years of life and continue to carry with you. Other negative thoughts are the result of a distorted view of events or simply unfulfilled expectations.

Albert Ellis, the creator of rational and emotional behavioral therapy, was firmly convinced that what affects us is not what happens to us, but our interpretation. These interpretations take the form of negative thoughts that cause us discomfort and, even worse, prevent us from finding a satisfactory solution to our problems since they often only serve to feed a vicious cycle of negativity. The first step to getting out of that loop is to know all the types of negative thoughts that can haunt your mind.

Are you a victim of these types of negative thoughts?

There are as many types of negative thoughts as there are people, but they can be summarized into eight large categories, easy to detect by the attitudes they generate.

1. **A permanent state of emergency**

Every time something happens, you take it as a total emergency. That reaction is because your amygdala is activated, and you can only see the alarm signal. A full-blown emotional hijacking occurs in your brain, triggering a panic reaction. By assuming reality as if it were a crisis, you react disproportionately. This type of catastrophic thinking leads you to exaggerate the dangers and underestimate your resources to deal with problems. This attitude can become very dangerous since it triggers a state of learned helplessness.

2. **The self-saboteur**

At the slightest difficulty, you automatically sabotage yourself. You take everything that happens personally and blame yourself for things over which you have no control. Your negative thoughts prevent you from thinking logically, so you punish and criticize yourself incessantly. As a result, every time a problem occurs, you lose self-esteem and self-confidence. This type of thinking makes you become your own worst enemy since you will constantly trip yourself.

3. **The extremist**

When something happens, you can only see the extremes. This type of negative thinking, also called dichotomous, makes you see the world in black and white, all or nothing, without a middle ground. It will be difficult for you to find a good solution by forgetting about the range of gray and intermediate colors. You will feel a lot of anxiety since you assume that any decision is a path of no return.

4. **The tagger**

Whatever happens, you label it in negative terms because you can only see the situation's dramatic consequences. The problem is that by placing those labels, you cannot see the possibilities that a situation can contain, so you close the path to its solution. This type of negative thinking can also cause you to label yourself and end up developing a very limited image of yourself and your potentialities.

5. **Tunnel vision**

When you have a problem, your vision is immediately reduced, like when you enter a tunnel. You only manage to see the negative things, problems, errors, and shortcomings. You fail to appreciate any positive details, possibilities, or strengths, so you fall into a downward spiral of negativity. This type of negative thinking is based on the phenomenon known as selective attention. In practice, it is as if you were wearing blinders and sunglasses to only see a very limited part of reality, missing the most important part precisely to find a solution.

6. **The generalizer**

When you have a problem, your mind wanders and begins to make loose connections between the present and the past events. These connections lead you to make wrong and negative generalizations, generally recognizable because words like "never," "always," or "all" appear. This type of generalization often leads to what is known as a "fortune teller's mistake," which is jumping to conclusions about something that hasn't happened yet, thinking that the results or consequences will be disastrous. Obviously, with each such statement, you lose a bit of self-esteem and strength, condemning yourself to a cycle of negativity.

7. **The impostor**

You constantly magnify the positives you notice in everyone else but downplay your strengths and talents because you tend to compare yourself. This negative thinking makes you feel like you are an imposter, and you don't deserve what you have. You are afraid that others will discover that you are not that smart, capable, kind, or bright, when, what happens is that you have a self-esteem problem. You are often the victim of what is known as "mind-reading," a phenomenon in which you presuppose what others are thinking.

8. **The superhero**

Your cape is always spread out; you strive not to disappoint anyone. You pride yourself on doing everything, whatever it takes. Your life is governed by "must" and "should" to the point that you completely forget what you want. The problem is that every time you realize that you can't save the world, your self-esteem plummets, and you experience extreme disappointment. It is one of the most damaging types of negative thoughts because you think in terms of "duties" and "obligations," allowing your life, decisions, and state of mind to depend completely on others.

The "Two" Sides of Doubting

Doubting is fine. It allows us to ask ourselves. It makes us reflect on our experiences. It helps us to make decisions, to weigh what we want or what we have done. Our doubts speak of our prudence and sometimes also of our humility in taking nothing for granted.

The maximum of some people is never to doubt. They envy those who take everything for granted and qualify them as extremely safe people. Doubting is healthy, even if we get on badly with it, and we love to dive between certainties. What is the difference between normal doubts and obsessive doubts?

Are doubts always "healthy"?

It seems it is not the case. And this is corroborated by some of the disorders suffered by patients with anxiety problems, where doubts have become the core of their lives, and far from helping them solve their possible unknowns, they immerse them in obsessive loops of which they believe they cannot leave.

What makes obsessive doubts different from the everyday doubts we all have from time to time?

Differences between normal doubts and obsessive doubts

- Normal doubts occur with direct evidence of the five senses and in an appropriate context.
- Normal doubts are resolved quickly once the necessary information is obtained.
- Normal doubts disappear once the person believes they have done what is necessary from a logical point of view, using common sense.
- Obsessive doubts exclude the evidence from the moment they go beyond the senses.
- Obsessive doubts increase the more you think about them.
- In obsessive doubts, the person never knows exactly what he is looking for. It is always a general "maybe."

Let's give some **examples of normal doubts**: "What will I eat tomorrow?" This normal doubt is given with **specific evidence/information** and takes place appropriately. Perhaps the person doubts what she will eat tomorrow because she wants to leave her food ready or already cooked tonight. Or perhaps tomorrow you will not have time to improvise and knowing in advance what menu to prepare will save you time the next day.

These doubts are also **easily resolved once the appropriate information is obtained** for it. In the example mentioned, this occurred when the person mentally plans the menu to eat tomorrow. By doing this, from a logical point of view, the person realizes that everything he could do to resolve the question is done. Doubt mentally elaborate the menu, and the doubt ends.

And what about **obsessive doubts**? For example: *"Will I have terminal cancer?"* (In a hypochondriacal picture). This doubt occurs **without direct evidence and in an inappropriate**

context. The person will go, for example, to the doctor repeatedly without having proof that they have any disease and will continuously check their body again without having information to justify it.

Even if logic and common sense tell you that you have no evidence of a serious illness, the urge to check will be stronger, and then the doubt will increase with the number of checks or reviews.

Through these examples, we can discover when the doubt is normal or when the doubt is pathological. When people immerse themselves, as we mentioned earlier, in obsessive doubts that are not appropriate or justified by the context in which they live, psychological intervention is necessary.

The objective is to teach people to differentiate between their normal and obsessive doubts so that they can **learn to tolerate the uncertainty** to which we all inevitably expose ourselves and to be able to understand what parts of their personality cause the person to become hooked on an obsessive doubt of diverse theme.

Negative Thoughts: The Power They Have Over Your Life

Negative thoughts are part of your internal dialogue, accompany you every day. Sometimes you are aware of them, and other times (most), you are unconscious. In this article, we will talk about the components of behavior according to cognitive psychology, how negative self- talk can cause psychological disorders, the most common characteristics and types of negative thoughts, and how to learn to identify and combat them. We leave you at the end of the article a document with exercises to try to start discovering your internal dialogue.

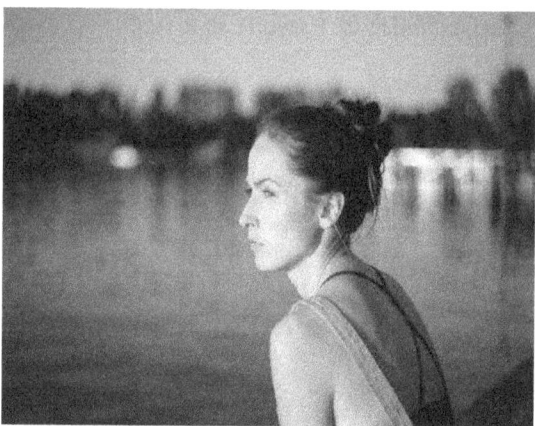

According to the Cognitive current, the thoughts are those that are under all psychological problems. Everything you do has three fundamental components: THOUGHTS, EMOTIONS, and ACTIONS.

The three are related to each other, and each one influences the other in such a way that when you want to change something, you must focus on modifying one of the three components so that the others "accompany you."

Everything you do has three fundamental components: Thoughts, Emotions, and Actions.

As the Greek philosopher, Epictetus said, "It is not what happens to us but what we tell ourselves about us." That is to say. You must be aware that you do not see reality, but you look at the world from your mental map, your representation, and your perspective.

Depending on how your internal dialogue is, this is how you will see the world. If you see the world under a veil of negativity thinking things like, "I'm worthless," "I'm very bad at this, "life is unfair, " "I'm unlucky," nothing ever comes out right," ... you will begin to generate negative emotions that accompany the thoughts and worst of all, that you will act as if you had really bad luck, or you were worthless or the world was a hostile place.

According to the law of Self-fulfilling Prophecy that defines Cognitive Psychology: if you think something, feel it, and act as such, in the end, you get reality to be as you had imagined it because you have caused it yourself. Suppose you think that your partner is unfaithful and that he is going to leave you.

In that case, you start to feel bad, sad, angry, you will begin to treat your partner with that anger and as if you were sure that he/she is unfaithful ... that situation It is very difficult for your partner to bear and ends up leaving you. Your partner has probably never been unfaithful to you, so your harassment made no sense, and in the end, you get what you feared the most.

Most of the time, we do not realize the power of our thoughts, what they can cause, and how they can change our lives. Only people who have managed to get out of the circle of negative thoughts and have started to think positively and behave in that way have been able to see for themselves how, at the end, when you want something good, everything is leading you to achieve it.

For example, you can start to think "I'm worth it," "I deserve a promotion," and that will generate a positive emotion and self-confidence that will make it more likely that you will talk to your boss, ask him for it, and that he will give it to you. I'm not going to fool you, I'm not saying that if you go to talk to your boss, you will get the promotion, but obviously, you have a much better chance of getting it than if you think you are not worth it or that you will never succeed in your job.

Why is it so difficult to change our internal dialogue?

Because practically all the negative thoughts we have been unconscious. They can be visualizations (mental images) or verbalizations (with words) that arise spontaneously. The psychiatrist Aaron T. Beck was the first to develop the most influential theoretical framework to address these thoughts and concluded that they are the most directly related causes of depression.

He also said that they are very difficult to change because they are part of our internal dialogue. We take them for valid and true without questionnaires; they are part of our being. Later it has also been proven that they are the most direct cause of anxiety problems, phobias, or obsessive-compulsive disorders.

Characteristics of Negative Thoughts

They are involuntary, thoughtless: you do not decide when you have them, but they arise spontaneously when something happens to you during the day. They cannot be controlled before they appear. We can only act afterward.

They have a pessimistic component: they describe your reality in a dramatic, catastrophic, sad way ...

They are distorted and superficial: they do not interpret reality rationally or objectively but conclude little data.

They are based on needs and demands putting a very strong emotional charge " *I need to pass that exam, or I will be a failure,* "*I have to get a girlfriend before the end of the year, or I will be alone* "

They are Specific: when we begin to feel depressed or very anxious, there is usually a very specific thought behind it, which we constantly repeat to ourselves ... What thoughts do you have throughout the day more times? ... " *he is going to leave me,* "*they are going to fire me,* "*I am sick, and I am not going to be cured,* "*I have no money* " ...

They are recurring: human beings have around 60,000 thoughts a day. Recurring thoughts occupy the highest percentage of those thoughts. What do you think the most?

They are credible: they do not have any solid argument to support them, but you believe them anyway. They are "absolute truths."

One test that you can put it to is to tell someone those thoughts or try to see them objectively. Normally the other person will not see it that much, or even from the outside, you see it as "ridiculous."

Chapter III: The Negativity Bias

Cognitive biases are psychological patterns that change the perception of information recorded by our senses, resulting in distortion, misjudgment, incoherent or illogical interpretation based on the information we have.

Social prejudices apply to prejudices in the identification and disrupt our relationships in our everyday lives with other people.

Cognitive Biases: the Mind Deceives Us

As an evolutionary necessity, the phenomenon of cognitive biases was born so that humans can make immediate decisions that our brain uses to respond agilely to certain stimuli, problems, or circumstances, which would be difficult to process all the information due to their complexity, and thus require selective or subjective filtering.

Cognitive bias can indeed lead us to errors. It helps us to decide more quickly or make an emotional judgment in some situations when the immediacy of the situation does not allow its logical scrutiny.

Cognitive Psychology is responsible for studying this type of effects and other techniques and structures used to process information.

Concept of prejudice or cognitive bias

Cognitive bias or prejudice arises from different processes that are not easily distinguishable. These include heuristic processing (mental shortcuts), emotional and moral motivations, or social influence.

The concept of cognitive bias first appeared thanks to Daniel Kahneman in 1972, when he realized people's impossibility to reason intuitively with very large magnitudes. Kahneman and other scholars demonstrated the existence of scenario patterns in which judgments and decisions were not based on predictability according to rational choice theory.

They gave explanatory support to these differences by finding the key to heurism, intuitive processes that are usually the source of systematic errors.

The studies on cognitive biases were expanding their dimension, and other disciplines also investigated them, such as medicine or political science. Thus arose the discipline of Behavioral Economics, which elevated Kahneman after winning the Nobel Prize in Economics in 2002 for having integrated psychological research into economic science, discovering associations in human judgment and decision-making.

However, some critics of Kahneman argue that heuristics should not lead us to conceive of human thought as a puzzle of irrational cognitive prejudices, but rather to understand rationality as an adaptive tool that does not blend in with the rules of formal logic or probabilistic.

Most studied cognitive biases

- **Retrospective bias or a posteriori bias:** It's the tendency to interpret predictable past events.
- **Correspondence bias or error in attribution:** It tends to overemphasize other people's rational reasons, actions, or personal experiences.
- **Confirmation bias:** It is the propensity that reinforces preconceptions to find out or interpret knowledge.
- **Bias in self-service:** It's the urge to claim more responsibility for success than failure. When we prefer to perceive vague knowledge as good for their purposes, it is also shown.
- **False consensus bias:** It is the propensity to judge that, among other people, your views, opinions, values, and traditions are more common than they are.
- **Memory bias:** The content of what we recall can be disrupted by memory bias.
- **The bias of representation:** When we conclude that anything is more likely from a premise that does not predict something.

An example of cognitive bias: Bouba or Kiki

The bouba/kiki effect is one of the most commonly known cognitive biases. It was detected in 1929 by the Estonian psychologist Wolfgang Köhler. In an experiment in Tenerife (Spain), the academic showed shapes to several participants. They detected a great preference among the subjects, who linked the pointed shape with the name "takete" and the rounded shape with the name "baluba."

In 2001, V. Ramachandran repeated the experiment using the names "kiki" and "bouba," and many people were asked which of the forms was called "bouba" and which one was called "kiki."

More than 95% of people chose the round shape as "bouba" and the pointed one as "kiki." This provided an experimental basis for understanding that the human brain extracts properties in the abstract from shapes and sounds.

Recent research by Daphne Maurer showed that even children under three (who are not yet able to read) already report this effect.

Explanations about the Kiki/Bouba effect

Ramachandran and Hubbard interpret the kiki/bouba effect as a demonstration of the implications for the evolution of human language because it gives clues that indicate that the naming of certain objects is not entirely arbitrary.

Calling the rounded shape "bouba" could suggest that this bias arises from the way we pronounce the word, with the mouth in a more rounded position to emit the sound, while we use a more tense and angular pronunciation of the "kiki" sound.

It should also be noted that the sounds of the letter "k" are harsher than those of "b." The presence of this type of "synesthetic maps" indicates that this phenomenon can constitute the neurological basis for *auditory symbolism*, in which phonemes are mapped and linked to certain objects and events in a non-arbitrary way.

People with autism, however, do not show such a strong preference. While the subjects studied scored above 90% in attributing "bouba" to the rounded shape and "kiki" to the angled shape, the percentage drops to 60% in people with autism.

The Halo Effect

The halo effect ("halo effect" in English) is prejudice or cognitive bias caused by the tendency to judge favorably specific characteristics of a subject by the general opinion that one has of him: human beings tend to generalize starting from a single attribute.

For example, imagine that you like a person; then, you will tend to qualify it with characteristics that will have favorable nuances even if we do not have relevant information about it. The Halo effect occurs daily, in many situations.

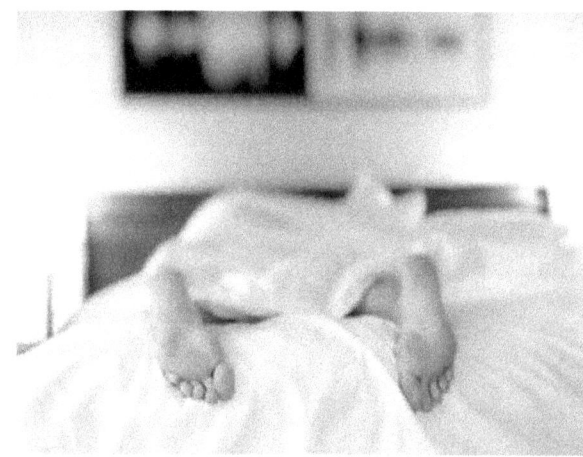

In the Halo effect, a specific feature is distinguished that is dominant, or that stands out from the start. This attribute causes us to attribute some distorted quality to it. It works interestingly with any type of quality if they are relevant to the judging person.

It is an effect that has a magic aspect, and that serves as an element that induces us to think a lot when we work for a brand, and we think about its target market group.

Its definition is Edward L. Thorndike, an American psychologist and pedagogue, a behavioral psychology predecessor. At the beginning of the 1920s when, in one of his studies for the army, he realized that in the evaluations of the officers to the soldiers, there was a high correlation in the positive and negative traits: this means that when the different traits of a person, most positive or most negative come out.

A combination of both is not usually given, as would be logical. In his study, Thorndike found a high correlation between physical attractiveness, intelligence, and character, something that later studies also corroborate. An attractive person tends to be perceived as generous and intelligent. Physical attractiveness is one of the most powerful variables in the halo effect.

This effect can have devastating results and tarnish opportunities that we facilitate or prevent those around us: we live in a world of appearances in which beauty is a passport that can make it easier for many people to achieve goals and be valued for a positive trait of his image, with a perfect smile, a way of dressing, while if someone does not fit that model, he is directly discarded for many things, including finding a partner.

Making value judgments is something natural to the human being, and we do it without bad intention. Its meaning is merely evolutionary since, in this way, we anticipate possible aggressions. These judgments are usually the result of social learning (family, friends, media, etc.), and through them, we will end up conditioning our relationships.

Several studies indicate that in just seven seconds, we form an opinion of what we are seeing. This value judgment conditions our expectations and our way of relating to that person.

For the social psychologist Solomon Asch, physical attractiveness is the quality par excellence that characterizes the halo effect. Physical attractiveness is the variable that most evokes the halo effect. Physical attractiveness gives people measurable information about the halo effect, and it is some characteristics of physical attractiveness that best evoke this effect.

These specific traits make us judge an individual's personality—many of these specific traits (for example, eye color, hair color, weight).

For example, someone who is perceived as attractive, due to a part of their physical traits, will also be largely perceived as generous or intelligent. Many studies have supported the role of attractiveness in evoking the halo effect.

A recent study revealed that attractiveness could affect our perception of that person's life, success, and personality. In this study, attractiveness was correlated with weight. People perceived as attractive were evaluated as friendlier and more honest. On the other hand, Harol Kelly's, in his theory of personality, affirms that the feeling we have of a person will influence the way we will see them on future occasions. We will also attribute qualities such as being friendly, supportive, emotionally balanced, sincere, affectionate, and professional.

In marketing, this effect is also a very interesting concept to consider. It refers to a cognitive bias whereby the perception of a particular trait is influenced by the perception of traits that occurred previously in a sequence of interpretations: when a brand adopts an elite athlete, an actor, a singer, or any other type of celebrity. Automatically, the brand achieves the Halo effect associated with the celebrity's positive image status, and consumers perceive it based on it.

Similarly, if you have an opinion of a product of a certain brand, you will tend to get a similar idea of other products of the same brand, even if you do not have objective data to make an assessment. Companies use the halo effect to their advantage is to use different techniques to generalize positive opinions towards their brand and minimize negative opinions. Here we tell you what companies do to make a good impression:

1. Create a product without competition: The best way to stand out in the market is to be the first to create something. Apple did it when it released the famous iPod. It was so successful that Apple computers also increased their sales. Here you can see a very clear halo effect. If the iPod is good, the computers of the same brand have to be too.

2. Link your image to that of a famous person: Surely, you have seen many examples of this on posters and television advertising. For example, many footballers appear in advertisements. Soccer is the most popular sport, and everyone knows that footballers make a lot of money. Therefore, any brand where a soccer player appears is emitting messages that give off glamor and sophistication.

In compulsory education classrooms, you also find the halo effect more than desirable. This is manifested in the famous "labels" that many teachers put on their students. It is a phenomenon that often happens unintentionally because we are all used to evaluating what is happening around us.

If you have figured out that a student is brilliant, they will somehow perceive that they are valued more. Therefore, they will try harder and, even if unconsciously, the teacher will facilitate a little access to good results without the student realizing.

This also happens when evaluating. When you are correcting an open-ended exam, it is known that the evaluation given to the first question determines how the others will be evaluated. Now, a teacher must be aware of this reality and act in the most objective way possible.

Halo effect on Human Resources

This effect also occurs in Human Resources, specifically in two areas: personnel selection and performance evaluations.

- **The halo effect in a personnel selection interview:** Falling into the networks of this effect is one of the most frequent errors in selection interviews, and it is that the first traits that we recognize in others influence our perception of it throughout the job interview. One of the aspects that most influences this effect is people's attractiveness, as we pointed out above. A person considered more beautiful or attractive is generally better valued, even if they have fewer skills or competencies than a person without special physical attractiveness. However, it is indeed proven that physical matters are not the only thing that can give rise to prejudices, whose result is to give more opportunities to some people than others. We also have to consider today the halo effect in selection due to social networks. Today, they are one more judgment element to choose the right candidate for a job and the curriculum vitae. Some studies show that more than 60% of companies use at least two social networks to meet candidates.

- **The halo effect in performance evaluation:** They are used to know the efficiency of resources to achieve the objectives of the different areas of the company. Performance evaluation is based on periodic controls through which deficiencies in the performance of resources are detected. During performance evaluations, a manager may err on the subject. The halo effect may appear due to the evaluation based on a single factor such as physical appearance or good behavior. Recent behavior determines the outcome of the evaluation, regardless of what the employee has done the rest of the time. In this case, the manager would very well evaluate an employee who has done something very good in the last week and ignore his previous behavior. An example, in this case of a negative halo effect, is the presence of prejudices when a manager tends to evaluate a worker worse because of their gender, race, religion, etc.

Halo effect and Devil effect

The halo effect and the devil effect are two sides of the same coin. These cognitive biases have their origin in our brains' tendency towards simplification, drawing conclusions through inertia rather than performing an analysis of each fact separately.

The devil effect ("devil effect" in English) or reverse halo effect is identical to the halo effect but in reverse: it happens when specific aspects of a person are judged negatively if the general impression of this is negative.

As for the example of the devil effect, we will refer to a historical figure like Mao Tse-Tung. Everyone tends to criticize this figure for having imposed a totalitarian regime in China. Still, few will appreciate the economic and social achievements that it introduced in their country (for example, it managed to make the population of China literate, from 15% in 1949 to 80% in 1970, it turned a poor country into a great world power) due to its bad image that we have in the West.

But can we avoid halo and devil effects? As with the rest of cognitive prejudices, they are not at all easy to avoid, although the best way to assess a specific aspect of a person is to ask ourselves, Would we think the same about this specific aspect if it were someone else?

In politics, if we perceive a leader of any trend as attractive, surely many people will consider that their way of doing politics will also have attractive nuances, which is very positive for that person. Perhaps knowing this, in the electoral campaigns just before the elections, some candidates try to show closeness, empathy, etc.

Examples of the halo effect and devil effect

There are countless examples of the halo effect and the devil effect. In marketing, the halo effect usually occurs in consumers who have bought a certain product and have been satisfied with the result, causing them to value the rest of the brand's products in a particularly positive way. This is one of the reasons for Apple's customer loyalty to its products.

As for the example of the devil effect, I will refer to an article in the English newspaper "The Guardian" that analyzes the devil effect in Hugo Chávez. The devil effect makes very few people value Venezuela's economic achievements in terms of health and education due to the general bad image that was had in the West of the figure of its president, Hugo Chávez.

***Warning:** With this example, I do not intend to defend a corrupt and economically disastrous government like the Venezuelan one. I only mean to offer an extreme example of this cognitive bias.

The Negativity Bias

The Negativity Bias is a psychological phenomenon whereby people pay more attention and give more weight to negative experiences than positive ones. Negative stimuli are more conspicuous and dominant, and responses to threats and unpleasant things are faster and stronger than responses to opportunities and pleasures.

Bad emotions, bad parents, and bad feedback have more impact than good ones, and bad information is processed in preference to good information. This phenomenon is so general and encompasses so many human experience fields that it can be considered a fundamental law of psychology. We will see examples of this bias in different areas and, in the end, the evolutionary explanation of it. I will quote the main conclusions of the studies without giving all the details of the same;

Psychology books devote twice as many chapters to unpleasant emotions as to unpleasant ones. In a review of 17,000 psychology journal articles, 69% of them dealt with negative issues, compared to 31% devoted to positive ones.

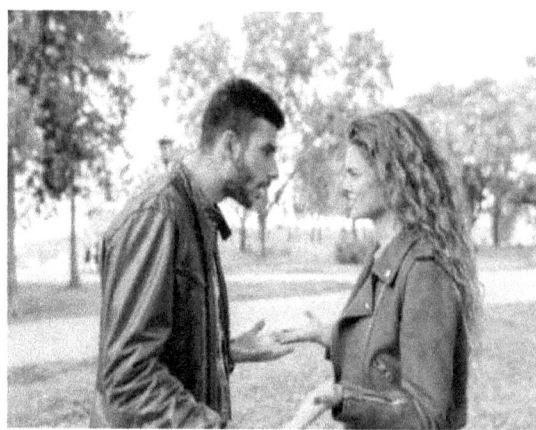

There are more words for negative emotions than for positive ones. Averill compiled an atlas of 558 words that describe emotions and found 62% negative and 38% positive. It seems that it is more important to label and discuss bad emotions than good ones. People also make more effort – and employ more techniques – to avoid bad emotions than to achieve good ones. Bad emotions are also remembered more and more effort and time is spent processing them.

People need to understand what happens to them, and the evidence supports that people think more and look for the meaning of things when bad things happen to us. When good things happen to us, we don't usually ask ourselves why they happen to us. We just move on. Threats in the form of aggressive faces are also better detected in various tests than neutral or pleasant faces. In the field of journalism, it is known that good news is not news.

The press is regularly asked to spread the good news, but these initiatives are often unsuccessful. The same happens in literature. Fiedler did a review of the history of the novels and said that no one had managed to write a successful novel about a happy marriage, whereas marital problems appear in countless novels.

In the field of human relations, we have many examples. In several studies of married couples, Gottman finds that negative affect reciprocates more and more strongly than positive affect, decreasing relationship satisfaction.

And it is not worth doing something good, to compensate, after having done something bad. Gottman proposes that positive and good interactions have to outweigh the bad by a ratio of 5 to 1. If this ratio decreases, the marriage has a high chance of failing.

The implication is that long-term success depends more on not doing bad things than doing good things. The same thing happens in the sexual aspect: a sexual dysfunction has more effect on the conjugal bond than a good sexual function.

McCarthy finds that when sexuality goes well in the marriage, it explains 15-20% of the couple's variance, but if the sex is bad or non-existent, it explains 50-75%. Bad sexual experiences, therefore, outweigh the good ones within a marriage. In one study, they tried to find out which factor most influenced the formation of friendship relationships in residence, and they found that it was proximity, closeness in coexistence.

But as they continued to study, they found that living close together increased the likelihood that two people would become enemies more strongly than the likelihood that they would become friends predicted. Since bad events are stronger than good events, increasing closeness produces more enemies than friends.

About learning, it is not politically correct to say so, but although textbooks say that reward is better than punishment for learning, there is no firm evidence. The works reviewed by Baumeister show, on the contrary, that punishment is more powerful for learning than reward.

About aversive conditioning, it can also be achieved quickly, sometimes with a single exposure. However, the conditioning of preferences with pleasant stimuli is usually much slower. The brain's response to negative stimuli is stronger at the neurological level, as shown by Smith's studies with the P1 potential, which show larger P1 potentials with them than with positive stimuli.

In how we react to things, we see that bad events have a more lasting effect and more intense consequences than good events. The effect of good events wears off more quickly. Lottery winners quickly return, after the initial euphoria, to their normal level of happiness.

At the same time, misfortune victims need more time to adjust to their fate because they continually compare their state to what they were previously, what Brickman called "The nostalgia effect." The discomfort of losing money is greater than the joy of winning it. That is, it hurts more to lose $50 than the joy of winning $50. The motivation to avoid losing something is much greater than the motivation to win something.

In the sexual field, there is evidence that a single trauma can have disastrous consequences for a lifetime. However, there does not seem to be the opposite of trauma, the "anti-trauma," a single positive sexual experience that produces benefits of a magnitude comparable to the damage caused by the victimization of a traumatic sexual experience. Having a good day does not influence how the next day will be while having a bad day usually influences how we feel the next day.

On the moral ground, knowing something bad about an acquaintance carries more weight, by far, than knowing something good. Bad reputations are easy to come by and hard to change, while good reputations are hard to come by and easy to lose. It does not matter that a minister visits hospitals 200 days a year.

If we find out that he does not pay social security to his assistant, he is lost and forever discredited. Since good behavior is frequent and expected, bad behavior is more revealing and important to know. To be categorized as good, one has to be good all the time, while to be classified as bad, one does not have to be immoral all the time, and therefore a single immoral behavior is already diagnostic (it is interesting that everything happens with intelligence otherwise: a very intelligent act causes a person to be classified as intelligent even if he later does various stupid things). Read that again.

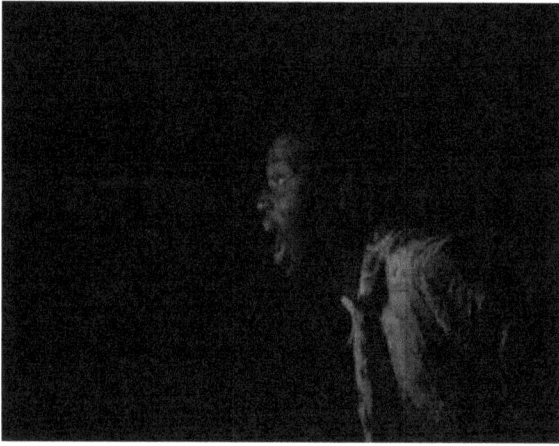

Once a bad act has been done, it is very difficult to wash it off with good acts. An initial impression based on bad moral acts is very difficult to change. As a curiosity, in a study, people were asked how many people would have to save their lives, someone who had killed a person to wash his act (he had to save them one by one and risking his life).

The result was that he had to save an average of 25 people. In one study, people were asked how many people would have to save their lives by someone who had killed a person to wash his act (had to save them one by one and risk his life).

On the subject of health, we all know that stress depresses immunity. Still, relaxation has not brought positive results of a strength comparable to stress in the negative aspect. In studies with medical students who were taught, relaxation techniques did not improve immunity.

It has also been seen that social support does not improve immunity, but that lack of support and loneliness does significantly worsen it. In a cancer patient study, optimism did not predict survival, while pessimism did predict mortality in the very young. Other studies have shown that pessimism, not optimism, predicts a good course of the disease.

By the way, some studies find that journaling about negative experiences, anxiety, depression, etc. improves immunity and physical health. In short, health influences our happiness when it is bad. If it is good, its effect is small or negligible.

The Negativity Bias and Evolution

Why is there the Negativity Bias? A pattern so widespread in almost all domains of our psychology, which also occurs in animals and young children, forces us to consider explanations that do not require language or culture.

Although other explanations have been proposed, it is inevitable to turn to evolutionary theory to understand where this characteristic of our mind has come from: that bad events have more power than good events is adaptive, responding to the world in this way promotes survival.

Both Rozin and Baumeister agree on this, although Baumeister dedicates more space to the evolutionary vision. Throughout our evolutionary history, organisms best tuned to respond to threats have survived and been able to pass on their genes.

A person who ignores an opportunity may regret it, but nothing terrible has happened. He may have other opportunities. However, the person who ignores the danger only once may end up maimed or killed. Survival requires special and urgent attention to bad events while dealing with good ones is less urgent.

Bad things, too, indicate the need to change something in ourselves. That is, they force self-regulation. Through self-regulation, the organism changes itself and adapts to the environment. The organism that rigidly adheres to behaviors that worked in the past may not solve the threats and challenges of the new times.

Looking at the phenomenon from this evolutionary perspective, we also understand why positive acts have a less lasting effect than bad ones. If satisfaction and pleasure were permanent, we would have no incentive to move forward, to seek more benefits.

The ephemeral nature of positive feelings would thus stimulate progress, which is adaptive. If bad feelings were to evaporate, people could repeat their mistakes at the risk of perishing. A further consideration in support of this view is that good carries a consistency in time and events that cannot be created by a single good event but can be destroyed by one bad event.

Good events need stability, linked to the asymmetry between life and death: the individual lives many years only if he manages to survive each day. There is no optimal experience of any kind that can offset the effect of failing to survive one day. There is no point in wasting time and effort, pursuing very good experiences at the cost of failing to survive.

Finally, to see what life would be like if the good were stronger than the bad, we could look at people who have congenital insensitivity to pain. These individuals experience more pleasant than painful sensations, but they often die young.

They suffer burns, amputations, and joint and bone injuries due to not realizing that they have to change their position, put their hand on the hot radiator, and trauma of all kinds. Subjects insensitive to guilt (psychopaths) would be another group rejected by the rest of society, losing the advantages that the group provides.

I think that everything discussed so far leads us to conclude that it is logical to expect that we are genetically predisposed to give more weight and attention to the negative. We thus see an example of what evolution can provide us to understand the functioning of the human mind.

The evolutionary vision allows us to lay the foundations for an adequate understanding of them: the answer to "Why?" It is not the last word, far from it, and on top of those foundations, there is a lot of taxonomic work and a lot of analysis to do, but we already have a cornerstone to build on.

Finally, I wanted to leave a very tricky question in the air that requires my approach. As you were reading, you probably have thought that living under the influence of this bias makes life not exactly very fair sometimes. How could we, if we want to build a better world, intervene to prevent some of the manifestations of this negative bias?

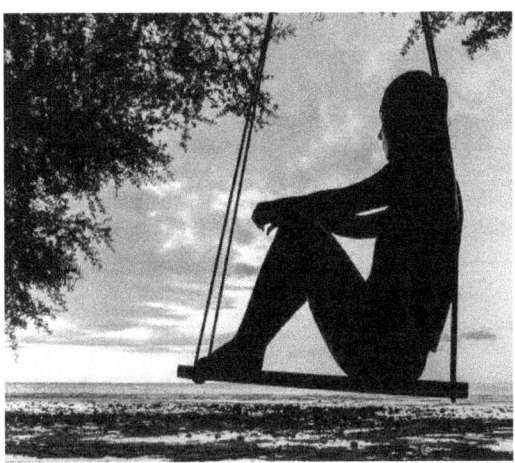

The rationale behind the negativity bias

A simple "good" is not enough if you want to convey enthusiasm. It must be expressed with more emphasis. A negative evaluation, on the other hand, does not need much more support. This is the so-called negativity bias. Recently, Christine Liebrecht of the University of Tilburg and her team have investigated how this 'linguistic injustice' can be compensated.

The study asked their probands to read a text about the conversation between person A and person B. They exchanged impressions related to their personal experience in a restaurant. Participants considered that the statement "The food was good" was less intense than the comment "The food was bad."

The same result was observed with the pairs of adjectives "smart" and "silly," "exciting," and "boring," "pretty," and "ugly." Negative words generally made a greater impression than positive ones.

But when the researchers stepped up positive adjectives (with terms like "wonderful"), the negativity bias decreased slightly. Participants even perceived a "very good" as more intense than a "bad." However, if they compared the expression "very good" with that of "very bad," the latter carried more weight than the positive phrase.

The authors are hardly surprised by the finding: generally, in interpersonal relationships, we express ourselves positively. A "good" is the starting point. For that reason, negative statements seem to have more force since they are rarely spoken in a social context. To this is added that negative comments would have a warning function that people do not want to ignore under any circumstances.

Negativity bias: how it influences our thinking

How many of us have cared more about being told something bad than having said something good? Human beings give more importance to what we see as something negative over what we consider positive or neutral.

Now we can assertively say that the negativity bias, or negativity effect, tends to give greater importance to negative aspects of a certain event, person, or situation. It is a fact of giving more relevance to negative stimuli than positive or neutral. This psychological phenomenon has also been called positivity-negativity asymmetry and has a significant impact on our daily lives.

For example, this phenomenon allows us to understand why people, when we meet someone new and learn about a negative trait about them, seem to focus exclusively on their bad characteristics. This would generate a negative first impression, which could hardly be modified in the long term.

It also explains why people tend to remember more those experiences in which some type of traumatic event has occurred or that we have not liked, over those that have been pleasant. We have insults more in mind than praise, we react more strongly to negative stimuli than positive ones, and we tend to think, more often, of the bad before the good that has happened to us.

Elements that make up the phenomenon

When trying to explain the negativity bias, the researchers Paul Rozin and Edward Royzman proposed the existence of four elements that compose it, which allow us to understand in more detail and depth how this asymmetry between the positive and the negative occurs.

1. **Negative power**

Negative power refers to when two events have the same intensity and emotionality but are of a different sign, that is, one positive and the other negative, they do not have the same degree of salience. The negative event will arouse more interest than a positive event with the same degree of emotionality and intensity.

Both Rozin and Royzman argue that this difference in the salience of positive and negative stimuli is only comparable, empirically, in situations involving the same degree of intensity. If a positive stimulus has an emotional implication far above another stimulus, in that case, a negative one, it is expected that the positive stimulus is better remembered in this situation.

2. **Negative inequality**

When an event, be it positive or negative, is getting closer in time and space, the degree to which they are perceived as positive or negative is different. A negative event will feel much more negative as it approaches compared to a positive event.

To better understand this: let's imagine two situations that involve the same degree of intensity, the beginning of the school year, seen as something negative, and the end of it, seen as something positive. As the beginning of the course approaches, this event is increasingly perceived as something much more negative than the end of the course, which is perceived as something that is progressively more positive but not so much.

3. **Negative domain**

The negative domain refers to the tendency that the combination of both positive and negative aspects results in something more negative than in theory it should be.

That is, the whole is much more negative than the sum of the parts, even if there is something positive between these parts.

4. **Negative differentiation**

Negative differentiation refers to how people conceptualize negativity in a much more complex way than positivity.

This idea is not surprising if we try to make an effort to count how many words are part of our vocabulary and are related to negative aspects. We would get a bigger list than if we focused on positive words.

It has been tried to give an evolutionary and biological explanation that people pay more attention to the negative aspects than the positive ones. Next, we will see what the evolutionary and biological bases behind the negativity bias are.

According to neuroscientist Rick Hanson, the negativity bias has an evolutionary character. According to him, this phenomenon is a consequence of evolution, since the first human ancestors learned to make intelligent decisions based on the risk involved in carrying them out. Those human beings who remembered negative events better and avoided them had a longer life expectancy than those who took more risks.

This behavior pattern is the one that survived, being passed from generation to generation, and now this bias is something common throughout the human species, given its great adaptive implication in the past.

The human brain was shaped to give greater importance to the negative aspects, pay more attention to them, and take into account potentially dangerous events for the individual's physical, emotional, and psychological integrity

Biological Bases

Studies carried out by the American psychologist John Cacioppo showed that **the negativity bias's neural processing implies a greater activation at the brain level** compared to the observation of positive phenomena.

This would be the biological explanation that would support why human beings pay more attention to the negative before the positive, going hand in hand with the previous point's evolutionary explanation.

Below we will see in detail some of the aspects observed about the negativity bias and its relationship with social and cognitive processes.

1. **Impression formation**

As we have already seen, the negativity bias has a significant influence on forming the first impressions of a person we have just met, which has considerable social implications.

According to the aforementioned, negative information about a person exerts a greater weight when preparing a general scheme of the same, that is, an impression, than those positive data that have been made known to us about that person.

Although positive and neutral aspects are known, the negative ones end up prevailing, influencing the formation of the impression, which is perfectly understandable if one of the elements of this bias is taken into account: the negative domain.

Another of the explanations given to explain the reason why the negativity bias occurs in social contexts is the idea that people believe that negative data about someone helps us to establish a reliable diagnosis about their personality.

Negative information is supposed to be somewhat more reliable than positive data, which may have been exaggerated or seen due to chance.

This often explains the intention to vote. Many voters tend to give more importance to the bad a candidate has done and avoid voting for him rather than giving importance to the desired candidate's information that turns out to be positive.

2. **Cognition and attention**

Negative information seems to imply a greater movement of resources at the cognitive level than positive information, in addition to having greater activity at the cortical level when more attention is paid to the bad than to the good.

The bad news, someone's negative traits, traumatic events, all these aspects act as a kind of magnet on our attention.

People tend to think more about those terms that turn out to be negative than positive ones, the large vocabulary of negative concepts being an example of this.

3. **Learning and memory**

Learning and memory are direct consequences of attention. The greater the attention focused on a certain event or phenomenon, the more likely it will be learned and kept in memory.

An example of this, although controversial, is how punishment exerts a greater weight on memory than does not reward it.

When someone is punished for having done something wrong, they are more likely to avoid engaging in that behavior which caused them harm, while when they are rewarded for having done something right, they are more likely to forget about it in the long run.

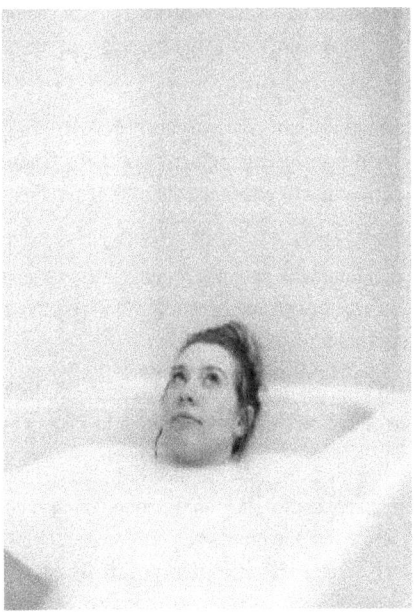

Although this should not motivate parents to punish their children more frequently for anything, it is interesting to see how the processing of negative events, in this case, punishment, seems to significantly impact children's education.

4. **Decision making**

Studies on negativity bias have also focused on how it influences decision-making ability, especially when risk is avoided, or loss is feared.

When a situation arises in which the person can either gain something or lose it, the potential costs, something negative, seem to outweigh the possible gains.

This consideration of possible losses and avoiding them goes hand in hand with the concept of negative power proposed by Rozin and Royzman.

Human beings tend to think about what did not go so well, instead of reflecting on the aspects that did. Hence, our pleasant and positive memories can be clouded by simple unpleasant encounters. This is what the negativity bias refers to the value we place on the negative.

Moreover, this is the bias that explains why traumatic events and negative experiences linger longer and seem to affect us more than positive ones. It seems that these more or less unpleasant experiences tend to become more intense in our thoughts. Let's go deeper.

On many occasions, bad news produces much more impact than good news, or criticism may even affect us much more than compliments.

In the book *The Buddha's Brain*, the neuroscientist Rick Hanson ventures an explanation, which has been endorsed by many other researchers, about the origin of the evolutionary character of this negativity bias.

According to Hanson, this negativity bias is a consequence of the evolution by which our ancestors learned to make smart decisions in high-risk situations. These types of decisions were what made them survive long enough to guarantee the next generation. They were a matter of life and death.

Thus, individuals who lived in tune with potentially dangerous events were more likely to survive. Over time, the brain structure adapted very slowly to pay more attention to negative information than positive information.

Different investigations seem to agree that this negativity bias develops in early childhood. Around the first year, babies' attention shifts from positive facial expressions to focusing more on negative stimuli.

In the studies carried out by the psychologist John Cacioppo on the neural processing of negativity bias, it has been found that the brain's response to negative sensory, cognitive, and motor stimuli provoke a much greater activation than positive events. Especially in the cerebral cortex.

As a result of the above, today, this negativity bias favors and influences our focus on the negative surrounding us, even when making a decision.

It also seems to greatly influence the motivation with which a task is completed. Curiously, a task that involves avoiding a negative experience motivates us much more than the motivation we put on a task when the reward is a positive incentive.

For its part, the evolutionary approach suggests that this is just a tendency that we have aimed at avoiding the damage produced by negative situations and that it is simply a way through which our brain tries to keep us safe and protected.

Although it seems that this bias of negativity has helped us to survive as a species, the truth is that in our day to day, it produces quite undesirable effects that should at least be known.

In addition to affecting our decision-making and the risks we are willing to take, this bias also seems to have a major impact on the way we perceive other people. In close relationships, it can lead us to think and expect the worst in others.

The negativity bias has consequences as diverse as those that make us more likely to give negative news more credibility than positive news. This type of news not only attracts our attention much more to them, but we also give them greater validity, although they may be false.

It also affects our values and ideologies and seems to have a lot to do with the tendency to cling to tradition and security in the face of ambiguous stimuli and changes that can be considered threatening.

As we can see, we should reflect on our tendency in most situations and take into account the presence of the negativity bias, especially if we want our decisions to be the most appropriate possible.

Chapter IV: Mind and the Unexpected Stimuli

Have you ever closely observed your reaction to anything negative around you? Let us forget the negative. Our reaction towards anything entails a fascinating process involving our mind and the information we consume. The information is called "stimulus" or stimuli in scientific lingo if more (usually more than one).

"We are at a loss of words to announce…", "It is with great sadness that…", "The new iPhone 12 will not feature a charging dock…", "World COVID-19 cases crosses 31.1 million." or "You are a dad now, Jim." Your reaction to these pieces of information may be positive or negative. In this chapter, we will specifically understand how the human mind functions to process good or bad information.

Let me give you some science. A group of researchers from the Faculty of Psychology of the University of Seville analyzed the effects of one of the most studied mechanisms in the control of the startle reaction: inhibition by pre-pulse. In their study, the experts used this tool to filter stimuli, facilitating the processing of relevant stimuli from the environment.

However, scientific results show that some of these filtering mechanisms, including pre-pulse inhibition, do not work properly in people suffering from pathologies characterized by alterations in the dopaminergic system, such as, for example, in schizophrenic patients.

The startle reaction is one of the fastest movements that humans make from a stimulus. This change in behavior, which prepares the individual for defense or attack, explains, for example, that we shout when they scare us, that we start running if someone is chasing us, or that, watching a scary movie, we close our eyes when starting a terrifying scene.

This involuntary response is produced by an unexpected sensory stimulus of enough intensity. But there are times when these reactions weaken. For example, the stimulus repeatedly appears when another stimulus of less intensity appears before the intense stimulus. The latter phenomenon is known in the laboratory as pre-pulse inhibition.

We can find a similar phenomenon if we think about the following situation: if we are at home with the door closed and someone opens it abruptly, the startle response will be produced. However, suppose before opening the door, they give a few gentle knocks. In that case, the shock is reduced or even disappears, says Luis Gonzalo de la Casa, professor of Basic Psychology at the University of Seville and coordinator of the excellence project *Dopaminergic modulation of inhibition pre-pulse for the presentation of novel and reinforcing stimuli in rodents and humans*.

Brain's Reaction to the Unknown

Pre-pulse inhibition is not only an informative measure of normal neurological functioning. Still, it can also offer information on psychological factors and physiological mechanisms in those psychopathological disorders in which the phenomenon appears altered.

In this case, it not only occurs in cases of schizophrenic patients but also patients with obsessive-compulsive disorders, Tourette's syndrome, etc.

One of the purposes of this line of research in which US researchers are working, and which they carry out in collaboration with researchers from the Department of Psychology and Neuroscience at Duke University in the United States, is to determine which are the neural pathways responsible for the coding of novel stimuli.

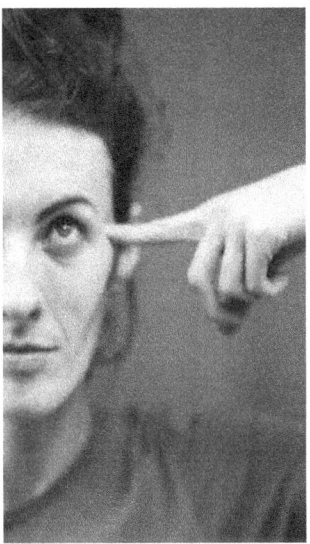

To this end, we propose the realization of two parallel experimental series, one using rodents as experimental subjects and the other with humans, in which the pre-pulse inhibition technique will be used as a behavioral index to evaluate the effect of the novelty on the dopaminergic system. says the person in charge of the project.

Why do we react quickly to fear?

An international team of scientists led by researchers from the Moncloa International Campus of Excellence (UCM-UPM) has shown for the first time in history that the human brain amygdala can extract information in an ultra-fast way in the face of possible threats that appear on the scene.

Thanks to their study, published in Nature Neuroscience, the researchers have obtained new data on how information travels between the visual and emotional circuits.

And is that the amygdala is a key structure in the processing of emotions within the limbic system. Unlike the cerebral cortex, the amygdala is located in the internal part of our thinking organ: "Its location is privileged; it is one of the most popular structures, connecting and receiving connections from various areas at different levels, and being able to trigger physiological changes or responses of the autonomic nervous system, "explains Constantino Méndez-Bértolo, a researcher at the Moncloa Campus of International Excellence of the Complutense University and the Polytechnic University of Madrid (UPM).

Despite this, its location also makes it difficult to examine it using the usual neuroimaging techniques.

The experts had the participation of 11 patients admitted to the Hospital Ruber Internacional who had electrodes implanted in the amygdala with which they carried out several experiments. The analysis of the tonsils of volunteers has discovered the first direct evidence in humans that this area can extract information on its own very quickly regarding possible threats or biologically important stimuli in the visual scene, before receiving the most accurate visual information neocortex.

The researchers found that the coarse information that the amygdala controls about the visual scene makes it sensitive to biologically relevant stimuli, such as the expression of fear of a person next to us, which also puts us on alert, prompting us to find out where it can be the danger.

"We started from the hypothesis that, if the amygdala presents an early emotional response, this will be greater for negative emotion and will occur whenever there are low spatial frequencies in the image since the information would come from the nucleus of the thalamus through neurons magnocellular, which do not transport high-frequency information," says Méndez-Bértolo, leader of the research.

During the experiment, the scientists observed that the amygdala had a very fast emotional response – less than 100 milliseconds to negative stimuli with low spatial frequencies.

"Thanks to this study, we can consider more important early and unconscious visual processing and the effects it can have on our body. It allows us to better understand why fear is often beyond our voluntary control," the authors clarify.

Bad is stronger than good: our brain is built with a tendency towards negativity.

- The negative stimuli produce more neural activity to positive stimuli.
- The responses to threats and unpleasantness are faster and stronger than the responses to the opportunities and pleasures.

- The negative events negatives are stored in long-term memory immediately. Positive events require us to actively think about them for a time ranging from 5 to 20 seconds to be archived in long memory. Furthermore, negative events are more easily retrieved from memory.
- We focus more attention on negative events than positive events.
- Having a good day does not influence how the next day will be while having a bad day does influence how we find ourselves the next day.
- Negative emotions, bad parents, and bad feedback have more impact than positive emotions, good parents, and good feedback.
- The negative information is processed with higher priority than the positive.
- Of the words with emotional content, 62% are negative, and 32% positive.
- We tend to think that someone who says negative things is smarter than someone who says positive things.
- It is more difficult for us to enjoy something if we know that it has a defect. A great car becomes a worthless car simply because it has a button that sometimes gets stuck.
- The negative events influence twice in our daily events that positive happiness.
- The discomfort of losing money is greater than the joy of winning it. That is, it hurts more to lose $100 than the joy of winning $100.
- Given this tendency, there is the theory of prospecting, which means that when choosing what to do, if there is a known risk, we are more likely to act to avoid harm than to achieve a benefit.

And you cannot blame all that on our education or society. According to research done on 3-month-old children, they process negativity in the same way we do.

The reasons for the predisposition to the negative

It is a question of evolutionary survival. Thanks to the fact that negative or dangerous things have been more important than positive things throughout human history, human beings have survived. The brain tries that you do not do anything new, that you do not change because if you are well like that, it does not care if you are happy.

The brain does not care if you fight with your partner if you are bad at work or short. The only thing that matters to him is that you survive, not that you live.

The brain is programmed not to change, but it has a capacity for change that we do not always use. And that is tremendously important for any age. The brain seeks routine and automatism to avoid taking risks because 100,000 years ago, such a brain was efficient. But not today. Today there are no more lions in the street.

Practical consequences of predisposition to the negative

The brain's negative bias inclines us to give more value to negative emotions: sadness, fear, worry, and anger.

Examples in different areas of life:

- In politics, the parties encourage you to fear the consequences of voting for the opposite party. Thus, for example, the left parties convey the danger that the right governs because it will cut social benefits. And on the other hand, the right-wing parties will divulge that the left will raise taxes if it comes to power.
- In the field of communication and journalism, it is known that good news is not news.
- In raising children, we point out the negative much more easily and do not value the positive. If one day we tell our children that they are failures, this will likely give them more value than a whole month telling them everything we love them.
- In a marriage or relationship, if you tell your partner that you love them very much a month once a day, but if one day you tell them that they are not as attractive as when you met them, they will never forget that.

The same is true if you tell your husband that he is charming even though he is fat. Do you think he will be thinking about how charming he is? Gottman, an American psychologist, known for his studies of couples, proposes that for a marriage to work, positive and good interactions must outweigh the bad by a ratio of 5 to 1.

If this ratio decreases, the marriage has a good chance of failing. The implication is that long-term success depends more on not doing bad things than doing good things. The same thing happens in the sexual aspect: sexual dysfunction has more effect on the marital bond than good sexual function.

When sex goes well in the marriage, it explains 15-20% of the couple's variance, but if the sex is bad or nonexistent, it explains 50-75%. Bad sexual experiences, therefore, outweigh the good ones within marriage

People react to negative stimuli more. Take an example of the workplace. Regarding criticism in the workplace, Cliff Nass, professor of communication at Stanford University, suggests that bosses, if they have to praise the employee, do so after the criticism and not before the criticism. When doing so after the critical criticism, our brain has entered maximum attention.

So instead of saying your house is very beautiful, but I don't like the neighborhood, it would be better to say I don't like the neighborhood, but your house is very beautiful.

Knowing something bad about a known person carries more weight in the ethical field, by far, than knowing something good. Bad reputations are easy to come by and hard to change, while good reputations are hard to come by and easy to lose.

Regarding health, in a study in cancer patients, optimism did not predict survival, while pessimism did predict mortality in the youngest. Other studies have shown that pessimism, not optimism, predicts a good course of the disease. In short, health influences our happiness when it is bad. If it is good, its effect is small or negligible.

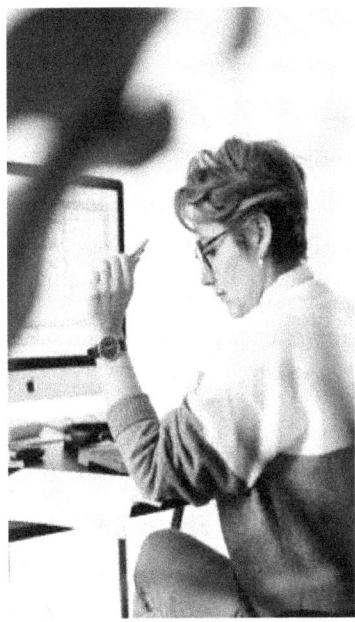

Studies done on rodents have shown that stress can harm the brain. Exposures of just a few days of stress, such as those we face in a normal Christmas season with the family, a community meeting, or at work, compromise the hippocampus's effectiveness – an important area of the brain responsible for reasoning and memory.

Weeks of exposure cause reversible damage to neuronal dendrites — branching protoplasmic extensions, or the little "arms" that neurons use primarily to communicate with each other and secondarily for cellular feeding. And months of stress can permanently destroy neurons.

We have already discussed discoveries that stress is only negative if you believe it is. One can usually deal with certain amounts of anxiety and self-imposed stress from the responsibilities we have decided to take on. You can understand it as positive stress because you have chosen it for yourself, it has a reason for being, and in return, you get results. Unfortunately, it is very difficult to apply this with the stress produced by people's negativity that we do not want to endure.

And it is that recent investigations of the Department of Biological and Clinical Psychology of the Friedrich Schiller University, in Germany, have discovered that exposure to negative emotional stimuli, of the type of pathological complainers, disqualifying, "guilty" and negative people in general, They have the same emotional reactions that are experienced when extremely stressed and, as with the stress response, the longer this is endured, the worse it is for the brain.

If it rains, it is bad, and if the sun rises too because the issue is to complain. Many people waste hours of their time trying to disqualify and see the fault in everything around them. They also go into states of anger easily if you disagree with their complaints.

You don't need to agree or agree with people who enjoy making complaints because they don't even want your opinion. They enjoy the process of complaining, and winding them up only further fuels their emotional hunger for attention.

The reality is that seeing everything black can become an addiction like any other. As the law of concentration says, according to Bernardo Stamateas, author of the book Toxic People: "The more you think about something, the more it becomes part of your reality."

Indeed, if for a long time you convince yourself that everything is wrong, for you, it will end up being so, and no one will be able to convince you otherwise. What's more, you may be mortgaging your health in the process of trying.

On the other hand, prolonged episodes of anger, such as those that toxic people suffer when you oppose them or in which they induce you to you, can wreak havoc on the body in the form of high blood pressure, anxiety, headaches, and circulation problems.

The investigations also show that even just a five - minute episode of anger is so stressful that it can jeopardize your immune system for more than six hours. All these problems can lead to more serious problems like heart attacks and strokes.

What's more, scientific research indicates that negativity is contagious, similar to a cold: the Framingham Heart Study, a one-of-a-kind project, which since 1948 has periodically collected medical and social information from thousands of people in Framingham, Massachusetts, found that a variety of habits and feelings such as loneliness, negativity or happiness seem to be as contagious as viral diseases.mHappiness turned out to be less social than sadness. Each happy friend increases a person's chances of personal happiness by 11%, while it takes just one sad friend to double an individual's chance of being unhappy.

"The more friends with the flu you have, the more likely it is to hit you. But once you have the flu, the time it takes to heal does not depend on their contacts. The same is true of happiness and sadness," said David Rand, an evolutionary dynamics researcher at Harvard to Wired magazine.

You already know them, you cannot save negative, aggressive, spiteful, or unhappy people, but they can sink you. And if your medical argument for keeping certain unbearable people away doesn't work, at least try to keep anger and stress as low as possible. The truth is, this applies to any extremely negative and unbearable person, there are those around every corner, and one cannot avoid them all. Therefore, I know that it is a difficult request, but with your health at stake. There is no choice but to try.

How Negative People At Work Affect You?

To create a great work culture, it is necessary to differentiate between honest, open, critical – constructive debate versus destructive, energy-draining language.

It is not enough to tell people "stop behaving like this" or "this can't be." It will be necessary to train, mentor, and coach team members in offering constructive criticism and positively expressing their ideas, to promote a change from "complaint" to "explanation" mode.

Some differences between these modes:

Those who complain	Those who explain
They do it to anyone	They do it before those who can do something about it
They do it with anger.	They do it when they are calm.
They present a monologue.	They create a dialogue.
They assume a bad intention.	They assume a good intention behind a decision or idea.
They point to another as guilty.	They accept responsibility for their own perception, attitudes, and behaviors.
They talk only about the problem.	They bring solutions, they offer to help find them.
They focus on qualifying others' (judgments).	They focus on observable behaviors (affirmations).

They talk only about what doesn't work.	They also include what does work.
They refer to how it impacts themselves.	They connect their concerns to a larger context.
They consider decisions to be personal attacks.	They understand that they are not personal, although they can affect them on a personal level.

The shift from a culture of complaint to a culture of explanation will not happen in an instant. It requires a group change of attitudes and leadership that models the expected behavior, reflected in their words and actions.

Identifying a Negative Person: the 19 Things Negative People Always Do

No one is always happy. Everyone has bad days. Sometimes extreme negativity can be avoided to improve your mood. In a recent article for Business Insider, Hillary White comments on the attitudes that unhappy people tend to have that they should immediately abolish. "If you work on positive thinking about yourself and others, you will be happy," she says.

1. **Worry about the things that cannot be changed.** "Negative people tend to think about what could have happened in life, but it is important not to worry about things that cannot be changed. You must learn from your mistakes and try to do your best next time. We can even be glad we made some mistakes, "says White.

2. **Give up when it's difficult:** Negative and unhappy people will always give up halfway when facing a challenge. It's easy to jump when something seems lost, but persevering, no matter the difficulties, almost always brings good results. "Giving up will make the person feel defeated. No matter how it ends, facing difficulties builds confidence," says White.

3. **Taking things too seriously.** Having the ability to relax and laugh at yourself and how absurd life can transform how you look at things around you.

4. **Not exercising:** Playing sports has countless mental and physical benefits. The more exercise you get, the better you will feel and will probably help you follow a healthy lifestyle. Leading a sedentary life will have negative health effects that will be noticeable in your mood and happiness.

5. **Focus on impossible goals.** "Having objectives is important; finally, it is the only way to do something. However, it can be tricky when these are impossible. Although we think it's good to reach the stars, people are always looking for unattainable goals. That is why they are always disappointed. The key is to set yourself small goals, which will make you feel fulfilled when you reach them," she adds.

6. **Eating foods that are not healthy.** Everyone has guilt-generating pleasures, and from time to time, it is good to permit yourself to eat them. For unhappy people, these licenses become a rule. Remember that healthy meals improve your mood, provide more energy, and are beneficial to your health.

7. **Not getting enough sleep.** Sleep is essential. Its quality and time are directly related to productivity and happiness the next day. "You may find that extra hour is a good idea, but a good night's sleep should be a priority," says White.

8. **Just focus on your weaknesses.** "We all have insecurities," says White. The key is to focus on the strengths and not the flaws. "Self-perfection is important, but negative

people tend to fixate on their flaws instead of worrying about having a positive image. Recognizing weaknesses is very different from letting them take control of our attitudes," he says.

9. **Spending too much time on social media.** "That is one of the biggest problems! Today people leave their entire lives online. First, that makes us spend a lot of time comparing ourselves to others," says White. It is highly recommended to have a good time away from the computer and have new perspectives on the day's activities. Negative people worry too much about how they appear on the internet, which will negatively affect them.

10. **Stay only in the comfort zone.** It's easy to want to stay in your comfort zone, where it is safest, and there are no risks. But spending a lot of time in that area means that great things don't happen. Boredom is a factor in unhappiness, which can be easily combated with new experiences. It is not necessary to leave everything and go parachute jumping. By trying new food or listening to music from a band you like, you can feel refreshed.

11. **Worrying a lot about the opinion of others.** "Negative people give too much importance to what other people think. But in the end, you can't please everyone, so you just have to be happy," she says.

12. **Always speak ill of others.** According to White, if you don't have anything nice to say, just don't say anything. Negative people try to bring down other people to feel better. But that never works.

13. **Overworking.** "Everyone deserves a day off. People who work hard often neglect their needs, and sometimes all we need to feel better is a day off," says Hillary White.

14. **Isolate yourself.** Although it may seem easier to isolate yourself from people in difficult times, spending time with friends and family is the best way to revive yourself.

15. **Never get out of the rut.** Happy people know that it is important to take a vacation, wear different clothes, and have a day to relax. Negative attitudes in excess make you forget that taking care of yourself is as important as taking care of others.

16. **Be comfortable.** "Negative people are happy to stay in comfort," says White. Staying in a relationship or job that doesn't make you happy creates a feeling of stagnation.

17. **Refusing to forgive.** Negative people tend to be vindictive and hold a lot of pain, but the peace and freedom that forgiveness will bring are greater than any sadness someone may feel.

18. **Avoid planning and organizing.** Disorganization can confuse our lives. Even something as simple as cleaning the room can restore order and help you gain a sense of control over

things. Negative people who avoid organizing are less prepared for the twists and turns of life," says White.

19. **Focus only on you.** Unhappy people think about themselves all the time. Treating others badly or always focusing on yourself and your problems can be detrimental to well-being and happiness.

The Negative of Positive Thinking

At the end of the extraordinary movie "The Life of Brian" is one of the most delusional and successful scenes I have ever seen. Many people executed and nailed to the cross to cheer Brian, the main character, against the terrible mistake that his sentence to die crucified supposes.

One of them, a character who reminds us of the Bible's good thief, begins to harangue the rest to tell them something about the good things in their situation while Brian looks at him stunned. The scene has an in crescendo where everyone cheerfully sings a song titled, "Always look on the bright side of life." Simultaneously, the camera reveals a stark panorama with dozens of beings punished to crucifixion in front of a mass grave.

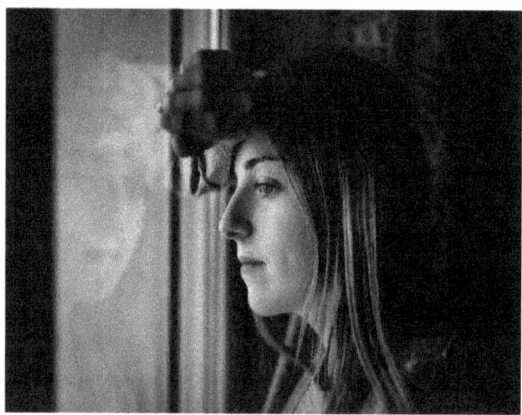

To this day, I feel that in those we are with everything that falls on us daily.

It seems that one is foolish if one does not take care to think positively.

A horde of inspirational leaders, coaches, and positive therapists excommunicate us if we dare to think negatively. You must be optimistic. You have to change it. You will get sick if you think that you will get sick and, even worse, you will create what you think about to burn in the fire of hell in life.

In the 21st century, we have reached positive fundamentalism.

Everything that is not that takes us away from success in life makes us worthy of dying on the scaffold. Life is great, but sometimes it hurts like hell. When you are bad, you cannot always think positive. Positive thinking, optimism, is born. It is not done.

Forcing yourself to optimize a situation is the best way to perpetuate suffering and is often the worst way to get out of a well. I have discovered that many people react very badly to the naive attempt to think positively when fear grips them or when life circumstances invite them to take refuge in the cave to lick your wounds.

Many people fall into the group that I call "Paradoxical People," that is, the more they try to encourage themselves, the more they become discouraged. The more they try to control themselves, the more they get out of control.

And it is that, when the bad vibes increase, our cognitive structure shows irrationality. Don't you believe it? Have you tried in vain not to feel afraid or to like someone you can't stand? The harder you try, the less you achieve your goal, and the more you start to feel worthless. We call that frustration.

Frustration undoubtedly appears when we find that our efforts to solve the problem do not work. When we see that we cannot do what we did with lower levels of concern or when we cannot follow well-intentioned indications from our environment. Negative thinking appears and remains, despite our efforts not to think. This is where we can change.

Where we can vindicate our mental capacities and take advantage of them in our favor, this is what I call an "efficiently negative thinking" and where despite the paradox, the fact of allowing ourselves to be negative leads us to a state of well-being.

Bullying: a Negative Experience in the Brain

The brain suffers the negative consequences of bullying if bullying occurs at a critical stage of life: 7 to 12 years. The impact can leave dire consequences on the victim's brain.

What is bullying? To describe it as such, at least one of the following elements must exist: repetitive bullying, physical violence, creating negative gossip, or promoting social isolation towards a person.

For the aggressor, bullying is not a random process. It is present in him, with a history of self-harm, irritability, constant anger, and intellectual immaturity, always looking for the funny justification of his victims' acts.

What factors favor bullying? Small school classrooms, with a negative school environment, ages under 16 years, an environment with a majority male population and a history of depression, low self-esteem, and social isolation in the bullies' home. No involvement on the parents' part in the problems of their children and the low educational level of the parents. In other words, the best teaching a bully can have is found in her own home.

Whoever bullies intend to annoy someone with repetitive behavior is trying to exercise control of social power. Men tend to bully directly, with violence, and by seeking to humiliate. Women often intimidate indirectly through gossip and stories.

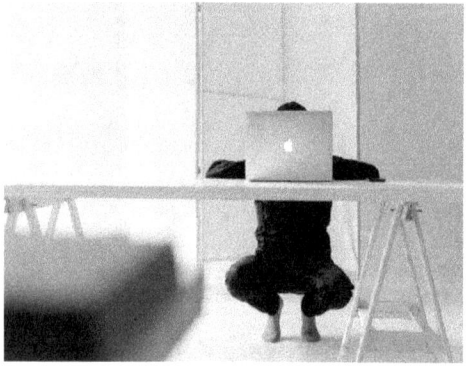

A recent article published in the prestigious journal Am. J. Psychiatry, in which a European population was analyzed through 58 years, identified that people who had a history of bullying have negative changes in life in their childhood. Consequently, the brain is the main organ affected.

Bullying favors the victim, the possibility of suffering anxiety, academic difficulties, decreased empathy and self-esteem, submissive attitudes, lack of confidence, and paradoxically there is also the possibility of favoring aggressiveness and the induction of provocative behaviors.

Victims of bullying have a common history: having an anxiety crisis, an antisocial personality, and favoring the decision to commit suicide.

In these patients, there are changes at the genetic level. The DNA undergoes modifications in key regions for its duplication or copying, the telomeres, structures related to the genetic material are modified or lost, with the consequence that some cells change their ability to adapt to stress, favoring early aging.

There is a propensity for the search for immediate satisfiers on the part of the regions related to pleasant events in the brain, so the onset of some addictions is favored.

Anatomical changes occur in the brain that affects the behavioral changes of bullying victims. Because aggression is constant, the brain enters inappropriate resistance codes. The brain amygdala triggers the clear majority of stimuli as negative: from apathy to irritability through crying.

The twist of the cingulate associate's inadequate interpretations of the faces. Consequently, the victims of bullying find it difficult to recognize others' pain and not interpret their own correctly. Psychological stress perpetuates itself as a critical stage of learning by the hippocampus.

Learning with pain and fear are the two main saboteurs in the school stage. This cognitive change is most difficult to forget, and in turn, the easiest to associate it with other experiences that have nothing to do with adult life.

At a neurochemical level, the decrease in serotonin in the brain is gradual and affects little by little, until it is recognized that depression is normal and every day. An over-activated brain amygdala and a diminished hippocampus are a terrible combination: a person who emits immediate behaviors with decreased ability to learn from mistakes.

A decrease in neurotransmitters serotonin, dopamine, and GABA condition depression and anxiety.

Coronavirus: the Loop of Negativity and Catastrophism

We are living in times of pandemic. Many months have gone by, and nobody knows when it turns into years. There is bad news all around us, and fear continues to rake in our nerves.

However, a sense of humor and relativization, understanding that we are not always in control and that the worst scenario rarely comes true. If it does, you can still get ahead: all of them are resources that even the most worried mind has at its fingertips.

Ruminating on our problems seems as inseparable from the human condition as breathing. We are programmed to detect difficulties and try to resolve them. The coronavirus pandemic has plunged the world into a paralysis (economic, social, and political). It has generated growing feelings of stress and anxiety in citizens (especially among those on the front line, such as staff in health centers or supermarkets).

If it is already complicated for someone whose anxiety has no real basis to control their emotions, what does psychology tell us when the uncertainty is not subjective, but nobody can predict how this situation will evolve?

You ask, psychology answers

The doubts that arise before this unforeseen and unpredictable panorama generate new questions capable of keeping the most stoic awake.

What if I can't stop worrying?

Faced with an unknown situation and when the person feels threatened, their internal alarm is turned on as a defense mechanism. The activation of our cerebellum and medulla oblongata, the reptilian brain where the human being's instinct and survival mechanisms, causes us to become more hypervigilant, restless, anxious. If it continues over time, it generates anxiety and emotional blockage.

When we are faced with a concern, we become obsessed with what occupies our mind because we do not know how to solve it. At the same time, physiologically, we somatize with reactions identical to an attack, and our pulse quickens.

In these cases, the best option is to be aware of the complete reality, that is, of what worries me and the "opportunities" that open before me. I am not able to see because I am immersed in obfuscation. In such a situation, we must balance the scale of reality, glimpse the good and the bad, maintain the psychological balance, not block ourselves, and facilitate actions according to the current moment, even if it costs us and the discomfort initially invades us.

But real people are dying, how can that not distress me?

Hyper information feeds back the blocking of our psychological defense mechanisms and restricts the real possibility of connecting with the present to find the best way to manage it. Being aware of the bitterest part of reality helps us maintain the guidelines that help us minimize damage. Still, it is necessary to know the real set and not be left alone with that part.

This is the message that has to resonate in the face of uncertainty. Respecting the limits stipulated at the social level and integrating them as one's favors keeping nerves and anguish under control: we feel that there are limits that must not be exceeded for the common good, which gives a feeling of security.

Is there anything I can do?

The most a person can do in a critical situation is to occupy themselves rather than worry. Staying installed in worry leads to blockage, inaction, increases the feeling of lack of control and lack of confidence and security. Taking care of the present means feeding positive actions that enhance well-being and calm, taking care of ourselves at all levels, and adding to the people close to us thanks to the affective bond we have with them.

The sense of humor helps us as an enhancing agent of well-being, unblocking our mind and keeping discomfort and, therefore, the immune system. It is another way of keeping a problem at a friendly distance to manage it better and not paralyze us.

By sharing something with humor, whoever receives it, and whoever provides it wins, the sense of cohesion is magnified and brings out the "taboo subject" in a less invasive way. That is, we will be taking care of others by facilitating them to connect with their humor.

What if I have been infected and am asymptomatic?

The protocol is clear. We must not skip it beyond having suffered symptoms or not. People who do not somatize the virus should not feel bad or good, since what happens exceeds their will and control. Although some live it with mixed feelings, with relief for not being in danger and turn with fear and worry about getting infected, if you haven't already, and about infecting your loved ones.

In this case, we return to uncertainty, not having answers, and being able to remain anchored in discomfort and worry. One has to choose between two positions: busy or worried. The first involves taking measures: taking care and taking care of yourself to minimize risks at all levels. The second position involves choosing the discomfort, with which the person disperses and cannot deal with the best way to face the present before him to remain installed in impotence and not be an active factor of change.

Eating, watching television, sleeping a lot, drinking, smoking, etc. It relieves me, but I start to worry if I have a problem

Everything that we use to channel anxiety in the face of an uncertain present will return, little by little, to its base level once we reposition ourselves. All of them are actions that were enjoyed when you had free time. The problem comes when the time has no limits or, due to circumstances, we have more free time available, and we still do not know how to manage it.

In a situation experienced as hostile, we use it as a defense mechanism that makes us feel better immediately, generating endorphins, the natural opiates in our brains. The problem comes when we must consume more of what makes us feel good at times, generating a collateral effect and the loss of control over it.

We have created greater tolerance for something that was once an exception and is now the norm. Suppose we feel that it has gotten out of hand. In that case, we have to be kind to ourselves and, in turn, put a "brake" for the present psychological well-being (reinforce self-control), and future (both for health purposes and for self-esteem, of physical and psychological well-being), which will only happen if attention is paid to what is done when it is done, and the purpose is identified.

Gaining awareness of the habits in which we exceed ourselves as an escape valve in the face of anxiety will help us to take responsibility and avoid generating discomfort in the long run if the lack of control is maintained over time of physical and psychological well-being), which will only happen if attention is paid to what is done when it is done, and the purpose is identified.

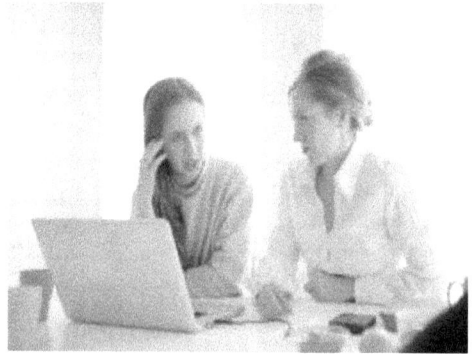

I can't stop worrying

We are unkind and uncertain emotionally. We are facing a time bomb. We are all suffering in the first person several duels at the same time. Since our reality has changed both personally and on a social level, without our having decided it, we feel that the reality that we had built until now has been taken away from us.

We have all felt lost without a clear direction. We live in the memory of the past from which we came, feeling longing, nostalgia, and sadness for what we do not have now. As mental health professionals always say, all the pain that we bring out can be handled from different angles to the pain itself.

Suppressing sadness, not crying it, or not expressing it will not make it go away. On the contrary, it will be feeding it within our internal silence, making it more difficult to manage and may crystallize into a future depression. You must accept the present, be aware of the total reality, not just the hostile part, and allow yourself to write with more or fewer letters that hurt us.

If you are not yet ready to share it with someone close to you, we can save it until the day you decide to do it or feel like you want to. Discomfort is not incompatible with having good moments, we must allow ourselves without guilt, as part of what it means to face the present, but unconsciously we will be choosing to put ourselves in a victim position, a situation from which we will make it more difficult to face the difficulties of the present.

This is the first step to win the battle against melancholy and sadness, and at the same time, activate the anger that is part of the same frame, but that will not take the leading role until the witness itself gives way. Anger will be the necessary counterpoint to activate that part of us that is asleep due to sadness.

Well-channeled rage activates action mode. At this point, we will be facing reality as such, emotionally and mentally, and we will be able to take the step of accepting the present psychologically without falling into resignation, or what is the same, being clear that accepting does not mean agreeing.

Chapter V: Positivity As An Imposition

Everybody wants to be happy. And what is wrong with that? A reader might ask. In principle, nothing. Although some experts – such as the Professor of Psychology at the Danish University of Aalborg, Svend Brinkmann – are beginning to warn that happiness may not necessarily be the appropriate response to many life situations.

Brinkman, who has dedicated a book to the dark side of positivity – Stand Firm: Resisting the Self Improvement Craze – says in his work that when something bad happens, we should allow ourselves to have negative thoughts and feelings about it. The author has even stated that although it seems natural to him that there are people of an optimistic and relaxed nature, we have reached a point where happiness has become almost a requirement.

The Swedish professor uses the work environment as an example. He says employee reviews often insist that employees focus on the positive and ignore their genuine difficulties, which Brinkman comes too close to an attempt at control of thought.

Meanwhile, Carla Barcelona, a health psychologist specializing in emotional work, warns of the dangers of positivity as an imposition or self- imposition: "These kinds of messages make you think that you always have to be well, or that it is always possible to be well. On one hand, it will affect your belief that those unpleasant emotions should be (even more) rejected. On the other hand, the moment you fail to be well, you can conclude that there is something wrong with you because they sell you that you can be well in theory, that you can handle everything.

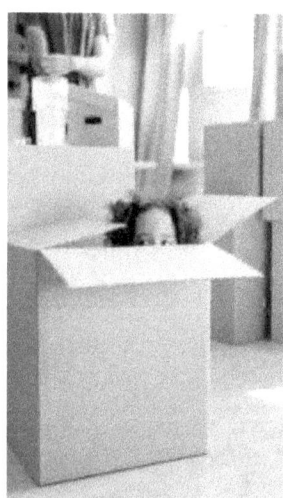

"It affects the belief that unpleasant emotions should be rejected and that if you can't be right, there is something wrong with you."

Barcelona also points out that labeling emotions as positive or negative already entails an implicit rejection of a full range of them. Precisely towards those that are judged as negative.

"It already happens simply because of the name we give them. You don't want something negative in your life, so it follows that those emotions shouldn't be there. The truth is that all emotions have a function and are necessary to adapt and relate to ourselves and our environment. Encouraging positive thoughts only increases this discrepancy, and that we have a longing (we can even idealize) those emotions that we consider positive".

Positive psychology is rooted in humanistic psychology developed by Abraham Maslow and Carl Rogers in the 1950s. However, it was not until the late nineties when Martin EP Seligman started talking about it and popularized a move that has resonated with numerous self-help books. Some could carry an implicit message that can be harmful to our mental health.

In recent years, different investigations have analyzed how emotions work and how they influence daily life, self-esteem, and well-being. These studies have shown that although positive psychology can help some people, it could be harmful to others; promoting feelings of failure, sadness, or even depression.

The danger of indiscriminately bombarding with messages such as "think positive," "being happy is a decision," or "everything happens for a reason" is that it can produce a feeling of guilt in those who have difficulties to be well.

So, is excess positivism dangerous? Carla Barcelona advises that "let's go simple, not positive. It doesn't matter if I'm thinking that I shouldn't feel this way, because what is happening is that I feel that way. If we understand that this is reality, then I can make a clearer decision about what to do with what I feel: take care of myself, support myself in people I love, or simply let myself be, for example".

The bombardment of positive messages can foster feelings of failure, sadness, or depression if you can't "be happy."

And is that positive messages regarding well-being can become a double-edged sword: "I can come to feel that I always" must "deal with my emotions, know what to do with them, and know their function. And not. Sometimes you just must leave yourself alone and stop demanding yourself to be well or deal well with discomfort. There are times when we get angry, others even explode, and the cause is that we are human, not robots".

Marc Bracket, founder, and director of the Center for Emotional Intelligence at Yale University denounces in his book Permission to Feel, how every day we suffer a subtle but constant invasion of messages such as, "you have to turn the page," "Stop thinking about yourself so much," "don't be so sensitive" or "you have to get over it." Bracket, who has spent 25 years studying emotions, says that "the irony is that when we ignore our feelings or repress them, all we get is that they become stronger."

A more useful vision for society is knowing that being bad is good. It is important to know each other emotionally and to know that we may not experience the same emotions as other people; after all, my reactions to my emotions may have more to do with the history and experiences I have with that emotion than with the emotion itself.

In this sense, a possible healthy posture could be to know that we are going to tend to judge and catalog our emotions, but that doing so does not prevent us from living with them, observing them, or relating to them in a more useful way for us.

Negative Emotions Have a Positive Side

Life is full of positive and negative emotions, but there is a huge inequality between them in practice. Society promotes the four winds of the former, such as happiness, gratitude, and compassion, while demonizing the latter, such as sadness, anger, anxiety, and guilt.

In this context, people have always sought to suppress negative ones because they associate them with violent behavior and consider them a breeding ground for developing deadly diseases, as scientific studies have revealed. For the British psychologist Tim Lomas, this classification is wrong. In his book The Power of Negative Emotions, he states that they are not as bad as they seem. Furthermore, he says that they are essential to achieve well-being and prosperity.

Lomas, an expert in positive psychology, carefully analyzes negative emotions in his book and demonstrates each one's value based on scientific evidence. Although he admits that they are unpleasant, he assures that they can be "potentially useful and, consequently, 'positive' if they are experimented in moderate doses and used wisely,".

Therefore, the book offers keys to take advantage of these types of emotions that usually bring information about aspects that are not going well in life. The important thing is to capture those messages and transform the negative into a force that helps build a more pleasant life. This is what the author says about each one.

1. Sadness

This feeling can present itself in various ways and regularly. Lomas says that normally people feel deep sadness when they lose a loved one or when a very precious object disappears. However, sadness's emotional pain has a protective effect, since these adverse circumstances allow the person to strengthen themselves, heal their wounds, and take the necessary impulse to move forward.

Neurobiologists associate it with hibernation because just as some animals protect themselves from winter's harshness, sadness can work in the same way that an exfoliant cleanses and rejuvenates the skin. Also, "it helps to better evaluate people and make them see things more realistically. That is why crying can serve as a catharsis".

2. Anger

This primitive emotion, which usually produces violent reactions, results from everyday events such as heavy city traffic or more serious things, such as having suffered abuse. Lomas mentions two types of anger in his book for each of these scenarios.

The first has to do with the impatience caused by being trapped in a traffic jam, something that the affected person cannot do anything about. In that context, anger is a waste of energy. The second is related to more delicate things such as a love betrayal, and in these situations, it is justified to feel it, since it serves as a defense mechanism to reject that injustice.

Although several studies say that it is much worse to suppress this energy than express it, Lomas recommends doing it with caution and self-control. Only a fine line separates the constructive power from the destructive power of anger. But some research has shown that in its fair proportions, this emotion can help improve interpersonal relationships.

"You have to know how to take advantage of it to change and not to attack the other. Getting angry can serve to gain strength and motivate us to face problems with courage."

3. Anxiety

It is normal to be anxious. While it can be unpleasant on some occasions, on other occasions, it shows that a person cares about proving themselves in different contexts and setting goals along the way. It is, therefore, very useful to learn and improve.

For Lomas, it is an internal risk detector that has allowed human beings to evolve, be alert to danger, and eliminate threats from their environment. The author cites the example of astronaut Chris Hadfield, who, in his autobiography, tells how NASA tests its crew so that they know how to react to any emergency.

Hadfield is, in fact, a proponent of the benefits of negative thinking. According to him, it allows us to know how to face and solve any problem in space and daily life. "Feeling anxiety should not be seen as a failure but as a way to get out of the comfort zone. It is much better to be concerned than to be complacent".

4. Boredom

Many stories of great artists and scientists whose great work or find came to mind amid deep boredom. Boredom, as tiresome as it may seem, can be a gateway to creativity and self-transcendence. Neuroscience is slowly corroborating its virtues. When the mind is wandering and does not have a fixed task, the subconscious can make new connections and even solve old problems.

Lomas found research by scientist Marcus Raichle who discovered the default neural network (RND), a set of collaborative brain regions that could be responsible for much of the mind's activities while at rest. Several neuroscientists claim that boredom plays a crucial role in the awakening of RND. That is why it is important to have total inactivity moments, without cell phones or television or books. The brain will appreciate it because it will increase "creativity and innovation".

5. Loneliness

There is a great paradox around loneliness. While people hate feeling alone, at the same time, they admit that sometimes they need to get away from everyone. But it is one thing to be lonely and another to be lonely. The moments of being alone are valuable because they allow self-insight and relaxation. "You need those oases of calm in which you can withdraw from the outside world and interact with others to feel peace."

In this topic, he recommends balance: not isolating yourself from the world but learning not to depend on others to be satisfied. This is a good way to gain autonomy and strengthen yourself to face any adversity. It also provides greater clarity about things and improves the quality of life.

6. Guilt

This feeling arises when someone believes that they were wrong or could have done things better. Although it is an emotion that, most of the time, make anyone bitter and can provoke self-destructive actions and thoughts, sometimes it is possible to take advantage of it. Lomas claims that people can use guilt to become better people.

"It is the opportunity to reflect and learn from mistakes. In this way, the motivation to grow and develop is found." The key is not to overdo it and punish yourself for any mistakes. No one is exempt from being wrong, he says, and the important thing is to transform this emotion "into repentance and compassion, which is very positive."

Enter Positive Thinking

Undoubtedly one of the keys that open the doors to success is positive thinking. And although it sounds very trite, many still have not managed to make it part of their lifestyle. They are still programmed negatively: some unconsciously and others due to the lack of self-determination to make the small change in frequency that gives us great results.

Positive thinking transforms our lives in all aspects, radically and positively. Thoughts are more than ideas or feelings. They are pure energy. Thoughts are biochemical and electrical impulses, waves of energy that penetrate time and space as far as we know. Therefore, each thought is an order that we give to the universe for better or for worse. What are you thinking about at this moment? Are you on a positive or negative frequency, do not forget that we are the result of our thoughts, of the emotions that we have felt, and the actions we have taken?

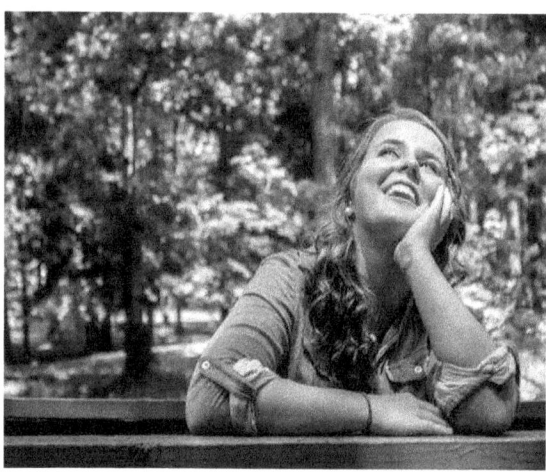

Therefore, you must be very vigilant of your thoughts to work in your favor helping you become the person you want to be, what you want to do, and what you want to live. The thought is like a seed that produces a flower and then a fruit. So, to reap the fruits, you must feed them with positive thoughts, emotions, and actions.

What are positive thoughts?

They are the only ones that allow us to accumulate inner strength and enable us to be constructive. Positive thoughts always benefit all situations without getting caught up in the external experience of a situation. Thinking positively does not mean that we ignore the reality around us and pretend to live in the unreal or pretend to be another.

For example, when we walk down the street, and there is a lot of garbage everywhere, saying that I do not see it, that I do not smell anything, is unreal. This is not what we mean by positive thinking. Thinking positively means seeing problems and recognizing their reality, but at the same time finding solutions to that problem.

Also, positive thoughts give us the feeling of inner contentment, and thanks to this, the expectations we have about the people around us decrease. What is extremely healthy for interpersonal relationships as they become more durable and harmonious. Another benefit of positive thoughts is that they are our best shield against diseases since if our body is balanced, we will enjoy excellent health.

Positive thoughts – to an optimistic attitude

This binomial is inseparable. If we are tuned in with positive thoughts by logic, our attitude will also be optimistic: the greatest protection against negativity in us and around us. With a positive mental attitude despite the problems that may arise in daily life, we will always remain peaceful, with great internal strength that will allow us to face challenges and find their prompt solution.

Positive Mental Attitude (PMA) is the right mental approach for every specific occasion. It can attract the good and the beautiful. The negative mental attitude (NMA) is the mental attitude of repels. PMA separates it from everything that makes life worth living.

The longer I live, the more I realize the impact that attitudes have on life. Attitude is more important to me than facts. It is more important than the past, than education, money, circumstances, failures, appearance, than talents and abilities. They build or destroy a business, a church, a home.

The remarkable thing about it is that each day we have the power to decide what attitude we will embrace throughout the day. We cannot change the inevitable. The only thing we can do is play the only string we have. I am convinced that life is 10% what happens to me and 90% how I react to it. And that's how it is for you. We are also in control of our attitudes. Finally, we have no choice but to continue working to eliminate those mental cobwebs.

Positive Thinking Culture

Every day we think. It is the natural exercise of our brain. Ask yourself how many of those thoughts in front of life, in front of circumstances, in front of realities, or front of people, are positive?

As per science, thinking positive is vital to keep arteries healthy. The natural flexibility of arteries is lost when we accumulate daily stress. One of the strongest drivers of stress are negative thoughts.

The way you think influences how you feel, which is why it is so decisive. If you learn to train your brain to think positively, you prolong life and make it fuller and happier.

It is about training ourselves in the return that positive thoughts generate to strengthen optimism and live better. Reality will always have limitations, imperfections, and difficulties. They don't change, but you can change your thoughts about those realities. There is the key, perhaps the most powerful decision to be happy.

The British statesman Winston Churchill said, "the pessimist sees difficulty at every opportunity. The optimist sees opportunity in every difficulty." That is the essence of someone who chooses to train their mind to think positive thoughts.

Choosing a positive or negative attitude towards reality is a personal decision in which the circumstances have nothing to do. If we are positive, we grow and act. If we are negative, we stop and regret big or small setbacks.

Positive thoughts are also products of our cognitive processes that increase our well-being and allow us to adopt an optimistic attitude. Besides, they enable us to act to attract beneficial events for us and perpetuate these profitable and satisfying ideas.

Robert K. Merton coined the term "self-fulfilling prophecy," which refers to our propensity to fulfill our predictions. For example, if we continually repeat that we are useless, we are likely to act as if this statement is true.

On the contrary, if we believe that we will achieve our goals, our chances of success will multiply. Thus, positive thoughts are one of our most powerful weapons to lead a full life and enjoy it to the fullest. We will discover this theory more, later.

Positive psychology

Psychology has been charged for most of its young existence to explore aspects such as "insanity." This discipline has had more influence on our negative aspects than on how to prevent them and how to find happiness.

Positive psychology is a fairly recent branch of psychology dedicated to studying our strengths, pleasant emotions, activities that are rewarding us, creativity, altruism, and other reasons why life is worth living.

Two of its main authors are Martin Seligman, especially known for his studies on depression and optimism, and Mihaly Csikszentmihalyi, a student of the state of flow (flow) and intrinsic motivation. Next, we will talk about positive thoughts from the perspective of positive psychology.

Positive Thoughts: examples

Currently, we can find endless examples of positive thoughts around us. For example, inspirational phrases are often shared on social media to help lift our spirits. In this section, we leave you famous optimistic quotes from well-known characters.

If you can't fly, run, if you can't run, walk, if you can't walk, crawl. No matter what you do, keep moving forward. – Martin Luther King, Jr.

The great discovery of my generation is that human beings can alter their lives by altering their mental attitudes. – William James.

The secret to happiness is not always doing what you want, but always wanting what you do. – Leo Tolstoy.

If you really want to understand something, try to change it. – Kurt Lewin

I have missed more than 9000 opportunities in my career. I've lost almost 300 games. I have been trusted 26 times with the winning shot, and I have missed. I have failed over and over again in my life, and that is why I have succeeded. – Michael Jordan

Having positive thoughts does not imply escaping from reality. However, unfortunately for our circumstances, we are primarily responsible for creating and directing our thoughts.

Viktor Frankl, a celebrated psychiatrist, and neurologist analyzed the search for meaning in atrocious and inhuman contexts. He was sent with his family to Nazi concentration camps. Only he and his sister survived. Despite the atrocities he witnessed, he also contemplated how some people maintained their desire to continue surviving and giving themselves the best.

Frankl developed logotherapy, psychotherapy based on the fact that we are all free and capable of finding our meaning in life. This can be achieved through our actions, our relationships with others, and acceptance of the suffering inherent in our existence.

How positive thinking works according to science

Millions of human beings live with a better attitude in the world. Personal work, psychology, professional coaching, and training in different disciplines contribute to their self-development and focus, manifested in greater well-being and assertiveness when solving problems.

However, some as many people live in disappointment, disenchantment, pity, and sadness. Why?

Science has found evidence of the power of positive thinking, not only from a purely "cosmetic" aspiration but a root transformer of the neural chains that we all have. Its proper use depends, to a large extent, the possibility of being more positive in managing life.

A study by researchers from the United States, Spain, and France reported that specific molecular changes in the body focused on mindfulness (also known as "Mindfulness") contribute greatly to an overcoming outcome. The study was published in the Journal of Psychoneuroendocrinology (P-s-y-c-h-o-n-e-u-r-o-e-n-d-o-c-r-i-n-o-l-o-g-y – I carefully Googled that).

Specifically, this study investigated the effects of meditation and positive thinking, mindfulness, and other techniques after a day of intensive practice. There were two groups: one of the people who meditated regularly, and another of untrained people, who were invited to do quiet activities, not specifically meditative.

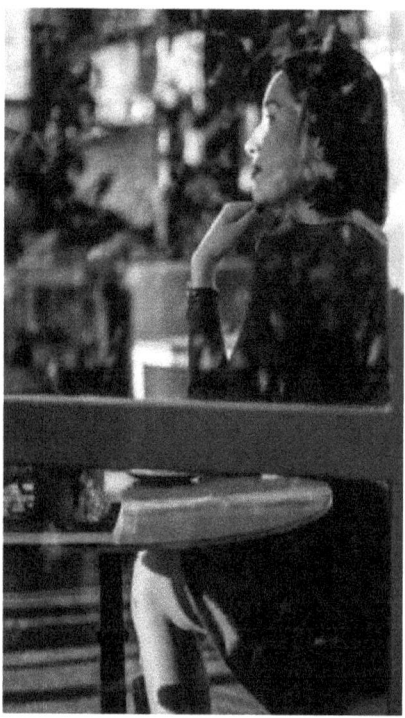

After eight hours of exercise, the first group showed genetic and molecular differences in their body, which included some altered levels of the gene regulation machinery, the reduction of genes that promote inflammation, and the ability to recover physically faster from stressful situations.

"To our knowledge, this is the first work that shows rapid alterations in the genetic expression of subjects associated with the practice of mindfulness meditation, among many other disciplines that help to achieve better living," says study author Richard J. Davidson, founder of the Center for Healthy Minds Research and professor of psychology and psychiatry at the William James and Vilas, University of Wisconsin-Madison, United States.

"The most interesting thing is that the changes were observed in the genes that are the current targets of anti-inflammatory and analgesic drugs," says Perla Kaliman, the first author of the article and a researcher at the Barcelona Institute for Biomedical Research, Spain (IIBB-CSIC - IDIBAPS), where the molecular analyzes were carried out.

Why are these results occurring?

The scientists stated that genetic activity could change according to the perception of each human being. This is directly based on their emotional intelligence ability, an attitude of life, and recurring chains of thoughts that each person brings, even unconsciously.

Dr. Bruce Lipton, who participated in the study, explained that "you can change the fate of cells by altering your thoughts." What does it mean? By changing your perception, your mind can alter your genes' activity and create more than thirty thousand variations of products for each gene. And he adds: "genetic programs are contained within the nucleus of the cell, and it can rewrite those genetic programs by changing your blood chemistry. "

What is this for? It means that we can change the results of our life if we change the way we think. "The function of the mind is to create coherence between our beliefs and the reality that we experience," Lipton said. "What this means is that your mind will adjust the biology and behavior of your body to fit your beliefs. If you have been told that you will die in six months, and your mind believes it, you will likely go to die in six months. This is called the nocebo effect, the result of a negative thought, which is the opposite of the placebo effect, where a positive thought mediates healing. "

To better understand that example: it is a three-part system. There is a part of you that swears that it does not want to die (your conscious mind); the one that, being conditioned by the part of you that does believe in what the doctor diagnoses you (your prognosis with the subconscious mind involved); a chemical reaction in the brain is set in motion to ensure that your body adapts to your dominant belief.

For Neuroscience, the Subconscious Controls 95 Percent of Life

What is your dominant belief? That is the one to which you have given all power. It may be recent, or it comes from your childhood. The result is the same: what you believe is what you become.

When Dr. Lipton was asked what happens to the part that doesn't want to die (the conscious mind), and if it can affect the chemistry of the body, he replied: "It all comes down to how your subconscious mind has been programmed. It is in this place where all your deepest beliefs are. And it is these that will ultimately cast the decisive vote in this choice between living or dying."

The chains of limiting beliefs

The chains bind and limit you; restrict your freedom. Limiting beliefs are chains that do not allow you to live fully. Here are some brief ideas to understand how the belief system works in any person:

1. All human beings live in situations over which we have no control.

2. We are programmed from before we are born with the beliefs of our parents.

3. For example, when we get sick, we are always told that we have to go to the doctor (this means that "you have to believe the doctor").

4. Many people who don't like going to the doctor got better just before going to the appointment.

5. This means that we also can have positive responses to wisely influence the outcome of our life.

6. If your negative beliefs dominate you, your life will be very challenging.

7. There are positive beliefs and limiting beliefs. It is the latter that determines your failures and non-beneficial situations for the results you seek.

8. If you exercise and practice positive thinking, gradually, over time, the chain of limiting beliefs will weaken, and only what supports your growth and development will be enhanced.

9. This requires constant practice, permanent surveillance 24/7, continued encouragement, and perseverance.

Cortisol, a hormone that generates stress, is secreted much more frequently in people with limiting beliefs until it invades their entire lives practically. From subtle levels to great manifestations of stress that even generate serious diseases, cortisol regulates brain activity. It determines how people will react "like the slaps of drowning" to get out of that situation if they want to.

Many people get used to living in a permanent state of negativity, anxiety, and anxiety. Over time, this becomes a liver disorder that is very difficult to get out of.

On the other side, we have endorphins, hormones that generate feelings of well-being, happiness, and pleasure. They are always present and ready to rescue from any pressing situation.

Science has determined that the continuous work of self-knowledge, deepening in the resolution of vital conflicts, stimulation of experiences of happiness and harmony, and any practice that helps to achieve that state, are appropriate tools to achieve a greater vital balance in all aspects; even recovering from diseases with a very poor medical prognosis.

"Our genes are very dynamic in their expression, and these results suggest that the tranquility of our mind can have a potential influence on their expression," says scientist Davidson.

Key: work on your subconscious beliefs

It is not about stopping feeling and being absent from the problems of the world and life: better yet, it is about being aware of what I can do for myself, to have a better quality of life, greater happiness, and well-being in all aspects, with practical awareness in every challenging moment that arises. This will allow you to exit more quickly and effectively.

Dr. Lipton explains, "the main problem is that people are aware of their conscious beliefs and behaviors, but not of their subconscious beliefs and behaviors. Most people don't even recognize that their subconscious mind is in play when the truth is that the subconscious mind is a million times more powerful than the conscious mind and that we operate 95 to 99% of our lives from subconscious programs.

"Your subconscious beliefs are working either for you or against you, but the truth is that you are not controlling your life because your subconscious mind supersedes any conscious control. So, when you are trying to recover from a conscious level – quoting affirmations and telling yourself that you are healthy – there may be an invisible subconscious program that is sabotaging you. "

Here you will find ideas for you to exercise at this point. As always, it is your choice: only if you do, will you have the benefit. If you do not want to change, continue as before.

1. Consciously work your thoughts.

2. For each negative thought, it takes between 27 and 33 positive thoughts to, at least, neutralize it.

3. Develop a positive routine.

4. Meditate or take quiet time to reflect.

5. Avoid busy environments.

6. Avoid people who are constantly negative and confrontational.

7. Take courses and seminars of different kinds.

8. Incorporate some physical exercise.

9. Disconnect your technological devices when you don't need them.

10. Discover your gift and abilities (for example, a hobby that takes you out of your everyday worries)

11. Nurture yourself with positive and stimulating readings, movies, and conversations.

12. What you resist persists: seek to experience flow with situations. Avoid reacting when you are in situations of extreme emotion.

13. Discover the little everyday facts that do you good: a look, a greeting, a hug, a smile.

14. Eliminate watching the news, especially before bed.

15. Be grateful when you wake up, during the day, and before falling asleep.

16. Listen to your body: always give good advice and signals.

17. Use the technique of positive affirmations: you will be surprised that most of the time, you have done it, but in negative.

18. Create moments of peace, even in your work.

19. Share your experience as you progress.

20. Ask for support from your environment.

21. Fix your gaze on the positive aspects of life. Far from stopping seeing everything challenging that always exists, you will better filter what is most convenient for you.

22. Observe your communication: if your vocabulary is full of negative, hurtful, misleading, and ironic words, it is time to become aware and put them aside. Replace them with ways of verbalizing whatever you want to say, in a way that is more conducive to yourself and others.

Being positive is a worn, discredited expression that has lost its authentic meaning until it has become an emotional simplicity. "It's time to be positive" is a resource for those who feel overwhelmed by a situation and try to hide it or those who intend to give lessons in "emotional culture" without mastering what they are talking about. "Being positive," "seeing the positive side," "seeing the glass half full," are rhetorical and hollow expressions, without content. We are going to try to clarify what is understood by positive thinking from scientific psychology.

The brain is a system that processes information, "it is not what it is, but what we think it is."

Information enters the brain from the sense organs. They are "inputs" that enter a relationship with the information stored in the memory of previous experiences and are encoded or interpreted based on that previous experience. The eyes look, the brain sees; the ear hears, the brain listens.

New information is first experienced on an emotional level (limbic system) as attractive or threatening. The cerebral cortex's reasons for the emotion experienced relate said emotion with previous experiences and interpreted the emotional charge's perceived situation. Thus, situations are not what they are, but how they perceive them, interpret them, take them, or live them.

Cognitive Styles or Ways of Thinking

We can talk about thinking behavior, what we do when we think, or our way of thinking or taking things, such as where we usually pay our attention, how we explain what happens to us, what usually worries us, what are our usual fears, in motor behavior we can identify habits or customs, thinking behavior also repeats actions that draw habits or cognitive styles, a way of taking things.

There are detailed people, others inattentive or distracted; Some are reflective, and others are impulsive, optimistic, and pessimistic, concerned, with humor, fearful, overly responsible, ironic. All of them respond to different processing styles that happen to them, to different cognitive styles or ways of thinking.

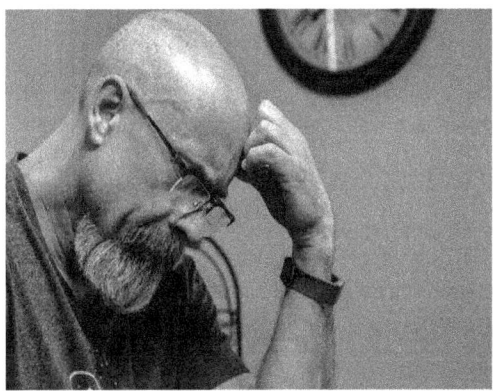

We feel how we think. We think about how we feel.

Thoughts activate matching emotions. Tell me what you think, and I'll tell you how you feel. It is explained at the neurophysiological level: internal dialogue or thought activates the autonomic nervous system and the endocrine system through the reticular system, shaping emotions.

A mind-body translation occurs, what you think moves biochemical changes shaping emotions. A thoughtful person, thoughtful, very responsible, perfectionist, who anticipates possible difficulties, habitually focused on the issues that concern him, lives with cognitive anxiety, suffers, suffers, does not enjoy, does not have inner peace, laughs very little. What we think has an emotional translation.

Emotions also activate internal dialogue. We perceive a situation as threatening, we feel the risk, and we activate concern, we anticipate the danger, generate mechanisms of the solution, and escape. If we feel attracted, we start an internal dialogue that convinces us to get closer, browse, get closer to the situation.

Thinking effective, being practical, versus thinking ineffective or being impractical

People move by goals or objectives. The athlete pursues performance; the worker, be productive: all people pursue emotional well-being. Being effective or practical means helping yourself achieve your goals. When illusions escape, you end up giving them up, possibly because of emotional clumsiness, making it difficult for yourself, ending up being your own greatest enemy.

Our head should be our best friend, who transmits us patience, confidence, renews our illusion, gives us clues on how to face and solve situations, brings us closer to solutions. Our head has to put our feet on the ground. It has to make it easy, and it has to lead us by the hand until we achieve our objectives. It is not the usual thing, but our head puts sticks in the wheels on too many occasions.

Our worries, excess of responsibility, fears, suspicions, perfectionisms, distractions, anger, discouragement, impatience, haste. They take us off the path towards our goals, even giving up our illusions, challenges, or dreams. Oneself can't become their greatest enemy, being their greatest source of discomfort and the greatest responsibility for their frustration.

Thinking that increases personal efficacy and enhances emotional well-being is identified as positive thinking. In contrast, the thought is a source of discomfort and takes away from the solutions or objectives we identify as ineffective, disturbing, or negative thinking.

Observe, identify and know one's cognitive style

Thoughts are not something hidden and inaccessible. We know quite well what happens when we think, what anyone does when they think about any matter. You have to talk about thinking behavior, what you do when you think. Thinking behavior is not observable, but it is manifest. We cannot observe what another person is thinking if they do not express it, but one is aware of what his thought is ruminating and what emotions it generates.

When we think we perform three cognitive actions, almost simultaneously:

- We put the **ATTENTIONAL FOCUS** on the matter we are beginning to think about. How long we put our attention on an issue, on what kind of issues we focus our attention more on, helps to be effective or make it difficult. The attentional focus can be under control, helping to gain efficiency.

- **WE PERCEIVE** the matter in our way, from our perspective or approach, from our experience, values, expectations, our emotional charge. In such a way, our previous experiences influence that we do not perceive what it is, but what it seems to us; We do not see reality, but what it seems to us. **We distort the facts from our emotional charge**. Observing the facts is not the same as giving free rein to impressions, assumptions, opinions, value judgments. Observing is not the same as interpreting or judging, the former being much more effective than the latter. Perceiving a situation from the facts or giving free rein to interpretations, beliefs, assumptions can also be under control.

- **WE TALK TO OURSELVES** (self-talk) based on how we perceive the matter and our cognitive style. Thought is an internalized speech, an internal dialogue, a self-dialogue. Speech or conversation with another person and thought have in common that they are **language**, they are speech. The difference is that the conversation tends to be logical and purposeful, while the internal dialogue is emotional or irrational, without any intention. In speaking with another person, you are prudent; there is an attitude of control, not to speak nonsense. In the internal dialogue, one can say real atrocities, unspeakable things, guided exclusively by emotions, without control, without passing the filter of the facts' logic. **Is it possible to put an order, introduce logic, have some control over the internal dialogue?** Clear!

There are two types of self-talk: one effective or positive, and the other disruptive or negative. The criteria to identify the type of internal dialogue are:

1) What type of emotions it generates if they are positive (illusion, desire, daring, trust, patience) or negative (anguish, anxiety, stress, anger, discouragement, hatred)

2) If it helps (effectiveness) or causes problems (ineffectiveness);

3) If they are supported by facts or reality (positive), or if they respond to distorting mechanisms of reality and self-deception (negative).

Observe how your cognitive style is, how you tend to think, what issues tend to hijack your attention, how you perceive or interpret, what you habitually ruminate in your head and the consequences of doing so. If it is easy for you to manage situations, make decisions, and emotions like an illusion, accompany, confidence, daring, your thinking is possibly effective.

If you tend to get confused, congested, feel anxious, overwhelmed, discouraged if it leads you to flee or escape from the situation. Your thinking is surely **ineffective**, impractical with yourself.

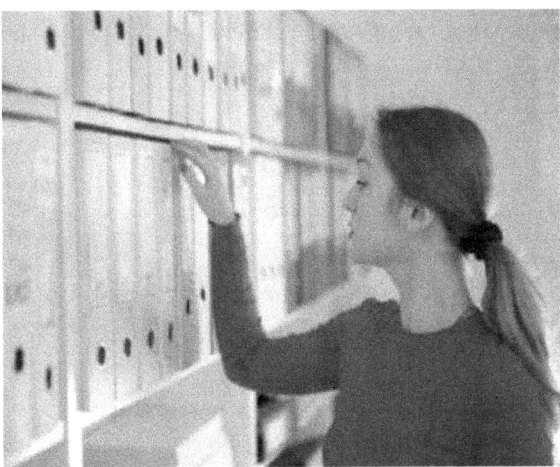

Much rhetoric is at odds with positive thinking.

Positive thinking is quite far from the use given to it in the street at a conversational level. "You have to see the positive side!" They say. Situations are not two-sided like the moon. Do we have to ignore the hidden side, less pleasant, more difficult, more painful? Is ignoring the unpleasant side to be realistic, or is it to fall into self-deception?

"Seeing the bright side" is insulting, a lack of respect in critical situations. All members of the same family being unemployed, not making it to the end of the month, suffering a terminal illness, the death of a loved one, what positive side do they have? None! Tell people who live in such a critical situation, *"you have to see the glass half full."* What empathy, what stupidity!

The truth is, any situation can be faced from acceptance and improvement, trying to understand what happened and mobilizing to manage the situation and overcome it feeling that it has been learned and evolved with it. The opposite means letting go, living at the mercy of the situation, and ending up being overtaken by it.

The most dramatic situation, such as death, can be faced from an attitude of acceptance and improvement, not without suffering grief. Understand death from the accident, illness, or the end of the life cycle, accept it because it is part of life, understand the pain and be willing to live with it until it fades, understand that life goes on, keep vital commitments, learn from what happened, recover inner peace. It responds to a realistic attitude, of overcoming, of managing pain and emotional discomfort.

On the contrary, not wanting to accept death, deny it, feeling that life no longer has meaning, inhibiting obligations and commitments due to pain, taking refuge in memories, falling into social isolation. It responds to an unrealistic, ineffective attitude that multiplies emotional discomfort.

No matter how difficult it may be, any situation can be faced and managed from an attitude of improvement, from a positive attitude. This is not seeing the "bright side." It has a positive attitude. A positive attitude implies realism, understanding, and accepting reality, to enjoy it if it is rewarding or to change it if it is difficult or conflictive. "See the positive side" sounds like self-deception, "do not see that aspect or aspect so as not to suffer."

Chapter VI: Theories of Positivity and The Law of Attraction

Who has never had this experience: You feel woozy, and even a little sick, when good news, a happy event, suddenly arouses all your energy. Suddenly you are in great shape, and you run across town to meet up with friends, or you can kill a day's work in an hour. But where did this renewed dynamism come from? By merely experiencing pleasant emotions? Therefore, could it be that pleasure, joy, happiness, positive thoughts are a factor in physical health?

The idea is not new. The psychologist and pharmacist Émile Coué, at the beginning of the 20th century, had even deduced a therapeutic method from it. He advised his clients to repeat aloud twenty times a day the optimistic message "every day, in every way, I'm getting better and better."

Years later, the American journalist and university professor Norman Cousins relaunched the idea by recounting, in 1979, how he had cured of a fatal disease thanks to a cure based on comedy films and vitamin C. But we had to wait a little longer for science to take an interest in the phenomenon.

For obvious reasons: "Medicine, psychiatry and psychology have amply shown how negative emotions and thoughts tense us up, tire us and, in the long run, weaken us. But, at that time, they were mainly concerned with pathology—the Positive Challenge.

Today, several therapies expressly appeal to the moral resources and dynamism of patients. Positive psychology properly strives to identify the psychic qualities that condition good health and promote the tools to develop them.

From the ability to meet one's material, emotional and spiritual needs, to the ability to overcome hardship, to the feeling of being caught in a positive "flow" that gives meaning to one's existence, these qualities have in common. 'address all levels of being, and insist on the dimension of sense, even of ethics. Just as we can ruin our lives brooding over problems, we can brighten it up by looking on the bright side.

Although several studies are beginning to demonstrate its effectiveness, positive psychology is not everything. It is tempting to perceive it as a resurgence of magical thought, a Coué method for idiots ready to believe that everything will always be better in the best of worlds if we are convinced of it.

In his latest book *La Fabrique du bonheur* (InterEditions, 2011), Martin Seligman, American psychologist, deplores that his discipline has been taken for a pseudo-science of happiness, a "happyology" advocating smiling, while it grants priority to the meaning and purpose to be given by each to his life. For him, good health does not rest so much on the feeling of happiness as on the one, more demanding, of development of all our potentialities.

For his part, Thierry Janssen does not fail to point out that optimism protects the organism. The link that unites happiness, health, and good humor depends on the deep meaning that we give to our life - a quest that cannot be satisfied by the only search for selfish well-being. Enjoying the benefits of optimism does not come without demands and responsibility. According to him, this requires prioritizing three mental attitudes that are the basis of our balance, three real pillars of our health.

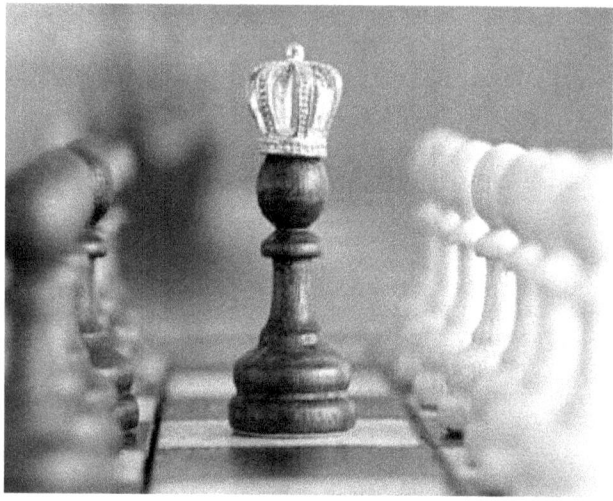

The fluidity. This is the primary asset. It promotes the flow of information and allows harmonizing the different dimensions of our being - a guarantee of good health. Lose your fluidity, for example, your ability to put into words your physical sensations and your emotions, and you risk causing or promoting the appearance of well-known disorders, often referred to as psychosomatic, such as stomach ulcers, asthma, eczema, or other chronic diseases.

However, fluency cannot be controlled – it would be like trying to force yourself to be natural. Let's follow the direction of evolution, advises Thierry Janssen let's start from the body. "You have to learn to untie it, relax it, to release the sensations and, suddenly, the emotions that are buried in it. And, only then, to put into words what we experience. Studies show that the simple fact of breathing deeply and moving your body rebalances the functioning of the brain, the balance between negative emotions (fear, anger, anxiety…) and positive emotions (joy, enthusiasm…). "

Concerning life as to oneself, it is an essential aptitude. But difficult: a good part of our personality was, on the contrary, forged in response to fears coming from our education or bad experiences. To be fluid, you have to learn to recognize your defenses, and the concerns behind them, things that no one likes to face head-on! How to do?

We can guess the answer: the body, of course! "Wilhelm Reich, an Austrian psychiatrist, and Alexander Lowen American psychotherapist have long shown that our fears and our defenses generate muscle contracture, physical restraint," explains Thierry Janssen. Hence the interest of adding a bodily practice such as yoga, tai chi, qi gong in any psychoanalytic or psychotherapeutic work. "

Consistency: Fluency and confidence require a sure consistency between intentions, thoughts, words, and actions. According to Thierry Janssen, life seems to demand this coherence to manifest and unfold fully. We see it at the biological level: as soon as everything is incoherence, life proliferates. If something inconsistent creeps into the system, it all falls apart.

Positive thinking, instructions for use

It is an attitude that is based on the principle that every individual has a rich potential that he must learn to use and develop:

- Combating the tendency to devalue oneself, anxiety and pessimism;
- By methodically training to mobilize towards clear and precise objectives, perceive the future with confidence, and creatively visualize the expected results.

The late interest of neuroscience

It was not until the 1990s that neuroscience began to investigate the mechanics of optimism. The data are accumulating: the placebo effect, spontaneous remissions, physiological benefits of laughter, the consequences of morale on aging, so many cases where optimism and pleasant emotions seem to play a positive role. Then, neuroscience highlights the chemistry of this process.

A new medical specialty is emerging: Psycho-Neuro-Endocrine-Immunology (P.N.E.I.) dedicated to body-mind relationships. Suddenly, in 1998, the professor at the University of Pennsylvania Martin Seligman launched a new psychological discipline devoted to the positive aspects of existence, called "positive psychology," and favoring the study of "fulfilled" individuals to identify them. Lessons applicable by the most significant number.

Optimists Live Longer, Healthier Lives

Countless studies prove it. One of the most significant, the famous Nun Study ("study of nuns" - "Positive emotions in early life and longevity: findings from the nun study," collective in *Journal of Personality and Social Psychology*, 2001) concerns a group of nuns sharing the same material conditions of existence, which makes it possible to distinguish the influence of psychological factors on their lifespans.

By studying cover letters written before entering a convent in the 1930s, psychologists at the University of Kentucky determined that the nuns identified as the most optimistic lived, on average, ten years longer than the less positive ones, and in better health.

For his part, the Dutch sociologist Ruut Veenhoven estimates that the most satisfied people live between seven and ten years longer than those who are less so after analyzing some thirty convergent studies. The power of morale on healing is less well demonstrated, studies sometimes contradicting each other – one showing the beneficial effect of support groups on cancer patients ("Effect of psychosocial treatment on survival of patients with metastatic breast cancer," collective in *Lancet*, 1989), another cannot confirm it ("The effect of group psychosocial support on survival in metastatic breast cancer," cooperative in *New England Journal of Medicine*, 2001). Excessive optimism, caution: imagining your success can lead to slackening your efforts and, therefore, failure.

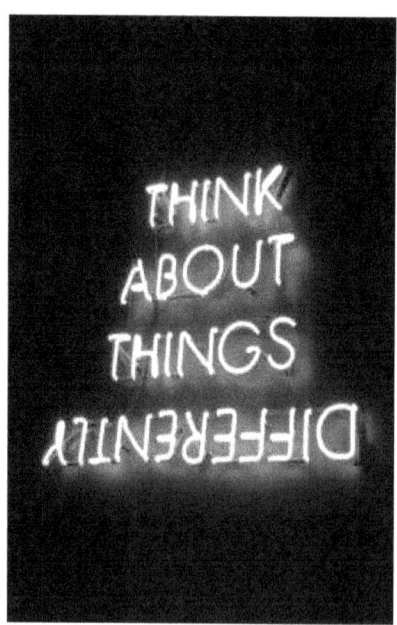

Positive Autosuggestion and Personal Development

Personal development and positive self-talk go together. Indeed, to move forward in life and personal development,

Therefore, working on oneself is necessary to achieve them, and our subconscious can help us with this. In other words, the subconscious is like a garden where the thoughts you sow in it grow. This subconscious is part of you and can serve you as well as serve you.

Therefore, depending on the thoughts that have been sown in it, consciously or unconsciously, the subconscious will act differently. Positive autosuggestion is the ability to interact with your subconscious through suggestions and constructive thoughts, thus nourishing your mind's garden.

Autosuggestion is the ability to interact with your subconscious through suggestions and constructive thoughts that feed the garden of your mind. – Dev-Perso

What is positive autosuggestion?

First, autosuggestion is a method that allows you, through your senses, to communicate with your subconscious. In fact, by sight and hearing mainly, you suggest to your subconscious the ideas and thoughts it should orient itself. The subconscious is very powerful because it directs life and attracts what it aspires to.

So, if you feed your mind negatively, you will be more prone to problems and hassle. On the other hand, if you provide your mind with positive thoughts, motivating, and inspiring, you will attract good and success in the coveted areas. Positive autosuggestion thus acts on the mind and the subconscious and changes its aspirations for a positive and optimistic goal.

Positive autosuggestion through emotion

For positive autosuggestion to be effective, think emotionally. Besides, move away from negative emotions such as fear, hatred, or jealousy and make room for positive emotions such as love, respect, empathy, trust. Whatever your thoughts and what you aspire to but feeling in it and find valid reasons following your values.

Positive autosuggestion through desire

Desire plays a vital role in your subconscious. Therefore, if you do not sincerely and strongly desire the object of your suggestion, the autosuggestion will have little effect. Consequently, you must frankly want to get what you think. Desire can also be nourished and maintained with work on oneself. Indeed, your mind has unsuspected faculties about the means it can implement to materialize what you covet (love, healing, wealth).

Positive autosuggestion by faith

When you focus on your goal, you have to believe it. In addition to believing in it, you must have firm faith that you will achieve this goal. This faith must be serene, sure, and ardent. Indeed, your mind and your subconscious will capture the message all the more as faith accompanies it. If you don't believe it, it won't work. Therefore, if you think it, positive autosuggestion can help you greatly.

Positive autosuggestion through visualization

When you practice positive autosuggestion, take the opportunity to visualize what you want. Indeed, your mind is receptive to what you see. Therefore, the external elements to communicate and interact with our interior go through our five senses. So, visualize what you desire. Imagine carrying out the actions you set out to do. Therefore, write down and display your motivations and goals and think intensely about it.

Also, be precise in the visualization. It will give wind to your spiritual mill. Effectively, it is the same principle as the subliminal messages for manipulating people or in advertisements. On the other hand, in this way, you influence yourself for your benefit!

How to practice positive autosuggestion?

Like a prayer, calm, close your eyes and focus on your autosuggestion. Therefore, out loud, distinctly, and in a sure and mellow tone, repeat what you wish. In other words, say exactly what you want. Remind yourself of why you want it by stating the reasons and the emotions that motivate you. Say that you have planned to move forward on a specific plan and know you can do it. Indeed, you can achieve this goal, you believe it, you know it, you visualize it.

Moreover, by dint of repetition, your subconscious will understand and print the messages. This means that it will work even when you are sleeping. In this way, it will help you find solutions and ways to achieve your goal.

Example of positive autosuggestion for someone who wants to lose weight and take care of their body

I want to lose weight, and I will lose weight this year. Because I respect my body and my health, and I want to take care of my body to feel better and be more attractive. Indeed, I can provide the necessary efforts, and I will provide them. Therefore, I have also planned a program that will allow me to achieve my goals. They are achievable, and I will reach them. I will even exceed them and go beyond what I thought I was capable of yesterday. Today, I have the strength and the state of mind that will allow me to accomplish what I want. At the end of the year, this is where I will be: (your goal). So be it.

Example of positive autosuggestion for someone who wants to become rich and free

Today I realize my financial situation, which does not satisfy me. To achieve freedom and not out of pride and vanity, I want to be rich and financially comfortable. Money will no longer be a problem for me or those close to me. I want it. I know it. I believe it. Therefore, I am already taking action to achieve this goal. Besides, my feelings and emotions are good, and this longing's finality will allow me to live the life I want. In other words, without having to work by constraint but by choice. This is why my choices and my actions are firm and thoughtful. I advance with confidence, and the path to wealth and freedom is more enlightened every day than the day before. I want to succeed, and I will follow. So be it.

Positivity, According to Barbara Fredrickson

Barbara Fredrickson, an American professor in the department of psychology at the University of North Carolina and author of Love 2.0: How Our Supreme Emotion Affects Everything We Feel, Think, Do, and Become, believes that the different definitions of emotion, although very diverse in content, agree that feeling can be conceptualized as a response composed of many tendencies that unfold in a relatively short time.

Emotion is distinguished from affect, which is a more general concept referring to consciously accessible sensations. Affect is one of the components of emotion but is also present in physical sensations, attitudes, mood, or emotional traits.

The emotion would be linked to personally significant circumstances for the individual (it refers to an object), while the effects are floating and with well-defined objects. Besides, emotions enter different families such as fear, anger, or interest, while affects simply vary over a bipolar continuum, which depending on the author, can be pleasurable.

The theory proposed by Fredrickson (2001, 1998) focuses exclusively on emotions as she defines them and more precisely on the positive emotions of joy, interest, satisfaction, pride, and love. For her (2001), positive emotions have an evident motivational impact because they engage the individual to interact with his environment to explore or control it. At this level, she believes that positive emotions are, like negative emotions, "specific action tendencies."

The specific tendency to act is a characteristic that is well spotted for negative emotions. For example, fear is related to the tendency to escape or anger to attack, to name just two examples. This tendency to action fits perfectly from an evolutionary perspective since the emotions would have allowed man to adapt.

Another complementary interpretation, which has been simpler to demonstrate from a biological point of view, lies in the fact that emotions have a psychophysiological activation function which prepares and supports the action of the individual by adapting, for example, the body running in the case of fear and focusing attention on certain types of stimuli.

The Fredrickson theory (2001, 1998) is in line with the evolutionary and psychophysiological perspectives of this tendency to action, inherent in positive emotions. The theory of the constructive expansion of positive emotions postulates that the five positive emotions mentioned above, although distinct, share the momentarily opening the repertoire of the individual's actions and thoughts, and this, to build his resources, be it physically, psychologically, or physiologically.

From this perspective, positive emotions acquire meaning for evolution since they allow species to perfect their adaptation to the environment. Although positive emotions can arise under hostile circumstances, they cannot occur when they are directly threatened. In certain situations, it is in the individual's interest not to seek openness but rather to be hermetic to pleasant stimuli and to prepare for the actions necessary for his survival. In other words, negative emotions have a direct adaptive function, but whose time horizon would be very limited, unlike positive emotions, which, in addition to a limited immediate adaptive function, would support the longer-term adaptation of the patient—the individual. Joy will create this constructive enlargement by encouraging play, pushing boundaries, and pushing creativity.

Interest encourages the individual to explore, seek new information, new experiences, and become personally involved in the activity course. Satisfaction forges constructive enlargement by inducing the individual to savor certain circumstances and integrate them directly into the self.

Pride promotes constructive enlargement by inspiring the individual to share their accomplishments with others, encouraging them to go even further. Finally, love which is conceptualized as the amalgamation of different emotions, creates the conditions of promiscuity and recurrence, which favors the discovery of the loved one.

Positive emotions can also prove to be an antidote to negative emotions by reversing the latter's actions. For example, Fredrickson & Levenson (1998) have shown that the cardiovascular impacts of negative emotions are canceled out when individuals experience positive emotions.

Another exciting aspect, promising in terms of research, is that some individuals use positive emotions in a resilient way and generate a positive spiral when they tend to be drawn into individual negative spirals such as depression. (Fredrickson, 2001).

Positive thinking is one of the main theoretical currents of personal development. It is a concept that appeared in the 1950s, and which was a real success with the release of the book "Power of Positive Thinking." It is a work that we owe to the American pastor and author, Vincent Norman Peale. Several million copies of this book have been sold, but it must be said that at the time, the ideas he developed were a subject of controversy.

Many people criticized the author for speaking much more to Christians. Nevertheless, the ideas conveyed have had enormous success, because even today, positive thinking is considered a fundamental tool for personal development. It helps to stay healthy, not only physically, but also mentally. It also makes it possible to increase life expectancy and to have more success in life, whether in the private or professional field.

If we consider positive thinking as a theoretical current of personal development, it conveys ideas that go in this direction. Indeed, positive thinking is quite close to the notion of optimism. It is a concept that encourages us to see the world more positively and see the bright side in every situation. It is an attitude that makes you feel better physically and mentally.

It has also been proven that people who apply positive thinking theories are happier and better than those who always think negatively. Thus, from the mid-20th century until today, several therapeutic methods based on positive thinking were created. They have made it possible for many people to find a solution to their problems and be happier.

Implementing Positive Psychology

Positive psychology is a theoretical current personal development. It is a discipline of psychology that was created in 1988. It was the idea of Martin Seligman, then president of the American Psychological Association. At first, many researchers considered this new discipline to be a pseudo-science. But today, we can say that it is a real industry, because every year, many training courses, internships, and coaching sessions are organized on the subject.

So, is this pseudo-science? It would still be necessary to succeed in agreeing on the real meaning of this expression. Even one cannot deny the existence of a certain number of human forces, which can help fight against various evils. These are forces that are, in fact, the best defense against mental illness. These include, among others:

- Work ethic
- Courage
- Perseverance
- Relational skills
- Honesty
- Optimism
- Hope

So, positive psychology is a science that was created from these different human forces. Its role is to prevent mental illnesses by promoting its virtues among young people.

If you are looking for another theoretical stream of personal development, consider the concept of life stages. It is a psycho-sociology that was developed around the 1970s. It is at the base of an idea of the researcher Daniel Levinson, but later, sociologists had to revise the stages described by the researcher. Ultimately, it can be said that Levinson's real contribution to establishing this stream of personal development is the "Dream."

According to Daniel Levinson's idea, the "Dream" is the influence of aspirations in the young adult's journey. Still, according to this researcher, the young adult must develop his dream, regardless of its nature. He must give it more clarity, and seek by all the means at his disposal, how to live this dream.

Neurolinguistic Programming

Neurolinguistic programming is a theoretical current personal development. It is a pragmatic approach to applied psychology. This was developed in the 1970s by two great American researchers: Richard Bandler and John Grinder. The goal of this programming is to model, on the one hand, the know-how, and on the other hand, the know-how of talented people in their respective fields of competence.

In other words, **neurolinguistic programming** makes it possible to work on the skills, attitudes, self-esteem, beliefs, and values of talented people. In this way, they can better transmit these talents to those who need them. Also, you should know that there are different levels of linguistic programming which are:

- The acquisition of personal skills
- The acquisition of interpersonal skills
- The "lifting" of barriers due to limiting beliefs.

Thus, thanks to this **theoretical stream of personal development**, improving one's self-esteem is possible. Neurolinguistic programming aims to improve in humans, autonomy, tolerance, mutual respect, surpassing oneself, etc. Even though this concept is considered a pseudo-science, it is sure that it has proven useful and effective for many people.

Auguste Comte and Positivism

Auguste Comte is the founder of *positivism*, a doctrine according to which the human mind cannot reach the essence of things and must renounce the absolute: this conception has had a major influence until our time. This philosophy, which gives precedence to the limits of reason over metaphysics, is also called scientism: man must limit himself to what he can know with certainty, thanks to science. Scientism is primarily based on Kant's critical philosophy, which denies man any metaphysical pretension.

The term "positivism" is a neologism admitted by the French Academy in 1878. Auguste Comte is considered the founder of positive science, although his influences and the concepts founding this science take their roots before the philosopher. Human progress is one of the fundamental ideas of the Age of Enlightenment, particularly in France.

Authors such as D'Alembert had already begun to theorize about the superiority of science. Still, it was Auguste Comte, who was to be the prominent standard-bearer of the positivist movement.

Comte was born in 1798 and died in 1857. He developed the positive sciences' idea during the first years of his life, then that of a positive religion of humanity. The principles of his doctrine will be taken up later in areas such as law and logic. Today, positivism may seem somewhat outdated. Nevertheless, Comte's doctrine on the Anglo-Saxon world and in Europe is not negligible, and the legacies of his doctrine weigh heavily in our societies.

Comte, positivism, and the law of the three states:

In the eyes of Auguste Comte, knowledge could not go beyond the sphere of scientific laws. Also, positive philosophy, which Comte designates his conception, is defined as a discipline having for object the coordination of the observed facts, without any pretension to go beyond the acquisitions of experimental science.

- Any investigation relating to the essence of reality is thus excluded from the field of research.
- This positive philosophy of Auguste Comte also bears the name of *positivism*, a term now widely used in everyday language, but which, in Auguste Comte, denotes the concept according to which the human mind cannot reach the bottom of things and must be confined to the sole search for the *laws of nature*, conceived as invariable relations of succession and similitude.

Positivism is based on the law of three states:

- The human mind goes first, according to Auguste Comte, through the theological form, a mode of explanation by agents holding a will (e.g., Zeus would exercise interventions that account for the apparent anomalies of the universe)
- Then by the metaphysical state, belief in entities or abstractions (the dormitive virtue of opium, for example)
- The positive state characterized by the abandonment of the "why" and the only attachment to the "how" in search of the applicable laws governing the phenomena.

This term of positive thus designates, in Auguste Comte, what is useful, real, and palpable instead of what is fictitious, chimerical, or imaginary.

This is the "law of the three states," conceived as the great law allowing to unify humanity's evolution. This law, which concerns the human species, in its approach to the positive stage, also appears real in the development of each individual: if the child believes in supernatural agents, the adolescent is a metaphysician, and the adult finally reaches the positivity.

We have headed to the final chapter. We are going to talk about the power of positivity, the direction which many of us can adopt. The Internet is flooded with articles constantly asking you to think positive, say positive, talk positive, walk positively, and alike. However, not much is conclusive or gives you a direction which can help you build the focus required.

The Law of Attraction

Many have heard about the famous Law of Attraction – which posits that our thoughts and emotions define our reality – but they are not convinced. They do not have enough evidence or a clear way to prove its existence.

However, in the same way, there are non-believers, there are many people convinced of this law, who claim that regardless of whether you believe in it or not, this law is ALWAYS in operation. For better or worse. I'm not necessarily going to tell you about the movie "The Secret." But if you haven't seen it, well you're not late.

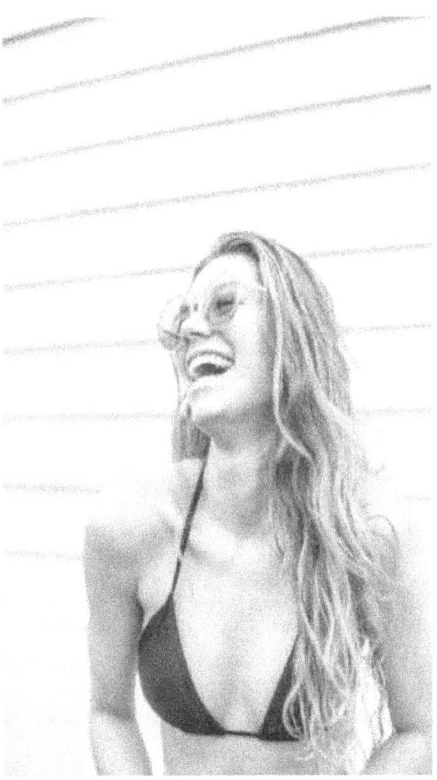

I do not deny that a lot of marketing and commercialization has been created with this term. But I think that perhaps the universe (seeing that we did not just open our eyes) put it in a commercial package because that does attract our attention as a society.

The universe has subtle moves to present us with clues. It is up to us to stay awake. At least, it is what I have learned in recent years, and it is surprising when you open your eyes to the Law of Attraction. First, you have to be clear and finish ACCEPTING that all things, desired and unwanted, are brought to you by this Law, one of the most powerful in the universe: the Law of Attraction.

Most likely, you have heard the sayings "the similar attracts the similar" or "what you believe comes true" (a belief is just a thought that you keep thinking). And although some of the greatest teachers in history have alluded to the Law of Attraction, never has it been explained in such clear and practical terms as recently.

The Law of Attraction is like the Law of Gravity. Believe it or not, if you jump off the roof of a building, you hit the pavement, whether you like it or not, with or without a Superman cape. So, we have to stop accepting the omnipresent laws governing this universe and how to make them work in our favor. A spiritual mentor that we listen to every so often on YouTube, and we have his books are the teachings of Abraham Hicks and his book The Law of Attraction. He can't put it any clearer.

With this knowledge of the Law of Attraction, you will understand almost everything that happens in your own life, as well as the lives of those with whom you are interacting; And you will discover how you can happily be, do or have anything you want!

Sure, this is not overnight. But it's like when you see a ship on the high seas going to turn. At first, you do not see any change of direction, you turn your eyes around for 10 minutes, and when you see it again, it is already in another direction.

But what is the Law of Attraction?

Well, in its beginnings, this Law was taught for the first time by Buddha when he proclaimed: "What you think, you will be. What you feel, you will attract. What you imagine, you will create".

Over time, the term "Karma" appeared, which today continues to be very popular and is sometimes used by society as a joke or misrepresented to annoy others. Karma is a central belief in the doctrines of Buddhism, Hinduism, Spiritism, and many others. It is not just one.

Karma is like "the law of cause and effect." In other words, the actions you have taken will come back to you sooner or later.

Simply put, the Law of Attraction is the ability to attract into our lives whatever we are focusing on. It is believed that regardless of age, nationality, or religious beliefs, we are all susceptible to the laws that govern the Universe, including the Law of Attraction.

It is the Law of Attraction that uses the power of the mind to translate what is in our thoughts and materialize them in our current reality. In basic terms, all thoughts turn into things eventually. If you focus on negative pessimism, you will stay under that cloud. If you focus on positive thoughts and have goals that you aim to achieve, you will find a way to achieve them with massive action.

That is why the Universe is such an infinitely beautiful place. The Law of Attraction dictates that anything you can imagine and hold in the mind's eye is achievable if you take steps in a plan to get where you want to be.

And what does science say about the Law of Attraction?

For decades and more, there have been many scientific experiments to demonstrate the Law of Attraction's power with cells and in other areas of modern medicine. In neurology and psychology, it has been seen how the mind can change the world around us.

It can no longer be doubted or denied that this Law has real effects on our lives and, while it is true that some scientists have doubts about it, they also have them about the law of gravity.

Over the last few years, the work of quantum physicists has helped shed further light on the incredible impact that the power of the mind has on our lives and the Universe in general. The more scientists and great thinkers explore this idea, the more we understand how important the mind's role is in shaping our lives and the world around us.

Raise your vibe, think, affirm, visualize everything you want, connect with love, with doing things well. The **Law of Attraction** shows that if you have thoughts of lack, poverty, bad temper, and complaint every day, you are only sowing what you will reap tomorrow.

Enter the Law of Attraction

Let's begin by illustrating what the Attraction Law means. It is one of the Universe's principal laws. The life of all beings that inhabit it is controlled by the creative force. Even if you are not conscious of its presence, it still accompanies you. Thanks to the power of thinking, attracting what you want into your life is possible. This makes it possible for you to think about something, interact with those actions, and produce energy towards the world, returning the same frequency about energy that you sent. You can attract your life's love, your soulmate, attract money, enhance your wellbeing, and everything you want. To implement the Law of Attraction, when raising your appetite, you must clean up your restricted beliefs in your subconscious mind and strengthen your attitude of complaint about a positive emotion. The Law of Attraction works to attract both good and bad, so it is necessary to keep vibrating in a consistently positive vibration tune or high frequency for this purpose. Believe it or not, it creates the difference between success and failure, wealth or poverty, health or sickness, love or loneliness.

You can get good things if you want good things, but you must still behave accordingly, not only wanting, but acting out of integrity. In the opposite, failure is inevitable and requires learning if your mind is full of negative thoughts.

Law of Attraction and Positivism

I want to help you be optimistic by doing this. In order to pay attention to this wonderful law in a very easy way, start step by step. So, you can imagine that the force of creation hits you in every way. Note, you are the source of the world, and as long as you have confidence and optimistic thoughts, even in times of adversity, you can construct everything.

When I saw **"The Secret"** on Netflix, it comes from the book of the same name on the Law of Attraction and the story of Joe Vitale, who even thought about suicide as a way out of the problems of his life under a strong depression He called me powerfully because now he has surprising luxury, it is a case of inspiration to be homeless to be a billionaire.

Beliefs and thoughts that you experience delaying or you do not believe that this may be true:

The Law of Attraction is a law, not a principle like gravity that works all the time, or you may detach yourself from the earth and objects in your house. Sometimes you think the law is not working, and they frustrate you, but it always works in the subconscious.

Test to Evaluate Your Connection With The Law of Attraction And Prosperity

I am going to ask you some questions based on a prosperity test by Randy Gage that I have even added doubts or fears that I have had or have been told by my clients in private consultations, look for a pencil and paper and answer yes or no to the following questions:

1. Are you afraid that your friends, family, or close ones at church will stop loving you if you become a rich person?
2. When you were a child, maybe they told you: "We are not rich, but we are very honest."
3. Depending on your religion, you may have heard that your life should be one of sacrifice and that your true reward will come in another life or plane?
4. Did you feel guilty when you started making more money than your parents, or did you somehow feel superior and started treating them like your children instead of your parents, questioning their financial actions?
5. Were you raised with a work-study mentality and not a business-studies mentality?
6. Did any of your favorite TV series from the 1980s onwards, based on fiction, portray the rich as bad, ambitious, and unscrupulous people?
7. Are you constantly suffering from aches and pains that doctors can't solve?
8. Have you become envious of people who own a good car, clothes, housing, luxuries, go to restaurants or travel?
9. Does being poor seem noble, romantic, spiritual, or philanthropic?
10. Did you, at some point, end an unsatisfactory love relationship and then start a similar one?
11. Do you use popular sayings or sayings frequently such as: "I am poorer than a rat," "poor but honest," "a bird in the hand is better than 100 flying", "you have to wrap yourself up to where the blanket reaches," to the 8 "guy?
12. You make excuses for not getting the money like: "You have to have money to have money," "you always need contacts to achieve things," "it costs a lot to earn money."
13. Do you think that life is a constant struggle, full of sacrifices and battles?
14. Do you like to raise pity in front of your circle, always saying that you have no money, you need help, and that you are very bad?
15. Can you meet your needs? Do you have a stable partner, family, and friends, but still think that life is taking its toll on you because good situations don't usually happen to you?

Very well, now I invite you to add your results. How many yays and how many nays?

Answers to The Prosperity Test:

- NO (between 13 and 15 questions), you have a strong consciousness about prosperity.
- YES (between 3 or more questions) you probably have some issues to resolve, blockages related to "worthiness and self-esteem " at a subconscious level. You are afraid to leave your comfort zone, and you are not radically happy. You know that something is missing, but you do not know what it is.
- IF (between 5 or more questions) you are probably in a stagnation cycle that does not allow you to advance, you make advances and retreats towards where you want.
- YES (to more than seven or more questions): you are on a downward path in your emotional and physical side, destroy the limiting beliefs, and start turning them into empowering beliefs, radically reprogram yourself.

This Law is surrounded by a great diversity of ideologies among human beings, notably determining our actions and reactions to an issue or situation. The type of collection of ideas or concepts that you keep ingrained during your life has led you to be where, and in the conditions, you are up to now.

Considering that everything is energy, with certainty, I tell you that according to this Law, you can attract many incredible things to your life! But for this, you must know how to use the secret. From within, you must be aware and convinced of what you want and how you will do it. Next, I will show you the Myths and Truths that have been handled around this Law. Check if you have any:

- **Myth #1: With only a positive attitude, you will achieve everything you want easily**

Truth – It is true that depending on how you express an attitude, you can minimize or aggravate your living conditions, but as you learn to live under the scheme of the Law of Attraction, it is a mistake to believe that you do not need to do anything more than that to attract what you want.

You want as much as you think positively about attracting something. It will not be enough. You must focus on knowing yourself and being clear about who you are and what you specifically want to achieve. Focusing on identifying what skills you have, your talents, the habits that you develop, having knowledge about what you like and are skilled, take that potential to exercise it.

Make it not become a work routine; instead, it becomes an activity that you love to do. To the extent that you first know how to be, then you can have.

- **Myth #2: By simply asking (decreeing), the Law of Attraction fulfills all your wishes.**

Truth – Here, that idea is taken from the phrase "ask, and it will be given to you." However, according to the Law of Attraction, synchronization is required on your part so that you can attract what you want in the future. It will depend on what think, say, and do, that together will generate the quality of energy to attract the good or more of the same, that is, what you do not want—besides, accompanying this with the constant implementation of known tools (thank, decree, affirm, visualize, etc.).

- **Myth #3: Applying the Law of Attraction takes me away from religion or spiritual beliefs.**

Truth – It has been scientifically proven that The Law of Attraction through MENTAL POWER exists and we all possess but were unaware of. It is how we can manage and/or modify important aspects of our lives in our favor. It has absolutely nothing to do with religion.

Some simply take passages from some sacred books to make similarities or interpretations that link it directly, but, The Law of Attraction is alien to any particular doctrine. Not by using this law in your life will you put aside your religious beliefs, you will only learn to handle your thoughts in a different way than what you did before, now you will focus or prioritize the positive side of everything.

- **Myth #4: To have a lot of money, you need to work very hard to get it.**

Truth – We usually carry this dissociation from our ancestors. We show a tremendous vulnerability to the belief that only a miracle can improve our economic condition. However, with the Law of Attraction, although it will not be an immediate event, you can do it if you propose it. A palpable example is Jack L. Canfield, the author of the book "Chicken Soup for the Soul," who set out to earn a certain amount of money and while he was in the shower, he remembered that he had written a book some time ago and began to consider the way to market it and not only did it meet its goal, but it surpassed it, now enjoying a privileged economic situation!

It is crucial to clarify these myths since when practicing the tools and not obtaining results, it is common to see that some people need this "external stimulus" to be able to believe in the effectiveness of the Law. Requiring others to share their experiences, and know what they managed to obtain, to know if they try to know it, apply it or not. But that is nothing more than a reaction from the scarcity of thought. I put this question:

How do you want to attract your desires and have the universe send them to you using (The Law of Attraction) if you are not interested in knowing it? From within you, not only the intention must emerge, but the "immovable faith" that motivates you to do so, and you can learn to use it.

Many people would rather live a life of lack than dare to believe that they can live a life of abundance.

The truth is that the universe does not respond to inertia, static, or passivity. It detects and flows through movement, which will originate with your actions. If you focus on something, this will expand. Your energy will oversee establishing synchrony with the Universe, and finally, you can co-create a dream future, which is the one you deserve!

How to Apply the Law of Attraction in Your Life?

There is a lot of work ahead of you if you want to live the life of your dreams, as I have repeated ad nauseam and countless times.

Perhaps some others who talk about the Rule of Attraction are convinced that it's almost magical. Still, I'm convinced that it's not something that is accomplished by daydreaming and without lifting a finger to reach it, to earn $2 million a year and buy a mansion on the shores of a paradise beach.

I am splitting my method of manifestation into several phases that I want to share with you:

1. **Define**

The first thing is to determine what you want, (as in almost anything in life). When I say "absolutely," it is because we can lose track of what that means with all the misinformation with which the media and the people around us bombard us on a daily basis.

Has it ever happened to you that you wanted anything for a long time, and you didn't enjoy the amazing and immense happiness you thought you were going to get when you finally got it?

This happens because we often imagine that we will also be pleased with the experiences or material goods that others have, thinking to ourselves: "If they are pleased to be millionaires, I will probably also be happy when I buy that huge house, get that desired upgrade or move to that awesome place."

2. **Emotions and Feelings**

You must first decide how you want to feel in order to prevent the above. Then make a list of the objects, persons, and interactions that make you feel that way at present.

My desire to experience the freedom to schedule my day as I wished was an example of my own, without being required to spend eight hours in an office, plus two hours in traffic, and, on top of that, having to settle for work redundancy. What I wished, though, was to be the owner of my time and my life.

That meant it had to work for me in my situation. I started creating my life plan after I figured it out, finding out what kind of company and career path I could establish to accomplish it.

For example, if what you want is to live by the sea, you should probably start searching for beach properties, find out their price, and then start thinking about the steps to take to get it and get into it.

You will also need to look for a job or options in the area that allow you to work from home or earn cash while travelling online. You just need to find out how every day you want your life to feel and then find out what kinds of individuals, experiences, and stuff will help you to feel that way.

3. **Plan**

Although many teachers and followers of the Law of Attraction suggest that we restrict the behaviour of the Universe by preparation, for me, a target without a plan is just a wish.

It is possible to raise $200,000 a year from home, but if you don't owe the world anything in exchange, you won't do it. If you do nothing else (with the exception of being frustrated), there is no point understanding what you want and wanting it so much.

For the rest of your days, you can daydream and lament about your reality, or you can prepare and work on it to achieve the life you want. I firmly believe that for what we want, we should ask the World, meditate on it and keep it present every day. But it's just half the work.

Determine the steps to achieve the goal.

Write points 1 , 2 , 3, and so on … until, if possible, 2023. And if the points 1.1, 1.2, and 1.3 have to be generated before moving on to 2, then so be it. In this life, your only task is to live it. So, why not do it and be happy in the best way?

Make a list once again: How much money do you need to earn? What job do you like and is it going to help you earn that amount of cash? Where would you like to live? What kind of people do you want to be surrounded by?

Answer all of your dream life's major questions and then work backward, finding out what smaller things you need to do first.

You must always bear in mind that it will not be easy to achieve your perfect life and that unexpected circumstances will also have an effect on your strategy. Put specific expectations out of your mind, therefore, which is why the next move is so crucial.

4. **Focus**

You've got to concentrate, people! Discipline beats inspiration, they say, and this is 100 percent real. Since you feel bad, sick, or sad, there will be several days when you don't want to work. It is nice to take time for yourself when you feel this way, but not to abandon your strategy for that.

In everybody's life, there will be moments that totally move the floor, but if you want something, you can't let that deter you. There's only one life, as far as we know, and we have to give it everything we have, to do the best we can about it.

Keep concentrated on your target and the steps you must take to accomplish it if you intend to move to that house on the beach.

Plan your budget, minimise costs, save on the move, figure out whether you can rent or sell your current home if you have one, determine how much you can spend on a mortgage per month, and check for local alternatives, etc. Focus on ONE thing at a time, mind you.

As much as the Universe is in your favor, you must act.

If you are fortunate enough to be presented with a great opportunity that is aligned with your desires and goals, but requires work and discipline, you must act!

Did you know that the book and documentary "The Secret" was inspired by the book " The Science of Getting Rich."

And while the book The Science of Getting Rich also mentions that our thoughts influence our reality and what we receive, there is a very important chapter not mentioned in The Secret regarding the Law of Attraction.

Do you know the name of the chapter?

It's chapter 12, and it's called "Efficient Action."

This is an entire chapter intended to make it clear that EVERY DAY, you must do what you can do from where you are and that you must do EVERYTHING you can. Give your MAXIMUM every day. Talk about the importance of making sure each day is a small success. To have the discipline and perseverance, so that every day you do everything that is within your power given your current circumstances.

If you give your maximum every day and do EVERYTHING that you should and could do every day, you will inevitably get what you want. Also, you will avoid saying the same as those about to die.

Quite different from the popular belief about the Law of Attraction that gives the impression that we should think or feel positively, have faith, and sit back and wait, don't you think? You can't find answers if you don't look for them. You will hardly achieve your goals if you do not go for them giving your best every day.

It is possible that when applying all this, "coincidences" begin to occur, and opportunities appear that you previously saw distant. However, if you do not take advantage of them, nothing is possible if you do not act and if you do not do your part by making the necessary effort when you require it.

Therefore, remember that this is one of the MOST IMPORTANT points regarding this famous law. Stay focused, focus on what you want, do everything that brings you closer to your goal, and you will see how you progress faster than you thought.

5. **Trust the process and have absolute faith**

Now that you've (1) cleared up what you want, (2) focused on what you do want to achieve, (3) worked on your limiting beliefs and negative thoughts, and (4) started to act, you should trust the process and have faith.

This is the time when you should get out of your comfort zone and dare to perform DARE actions aligned with your goals, even if you have no guarantees of results.

If you still don't have the necessary opportunities, keep upbeat, and try.

If you have absolute faith, then get ready to start receiving. Every day try to visualize the goal you want once it has been achieved.

- How are you going to feel?
- Who are you going to tell?
- How are you going to celebrate?

Take action with the absolute faith that you will receive what you want. Eliminate doubts and complaints. There is simply no room for insecurities, doubts, and complaints in mind full of faith.

Be confident that you will get what you want each day and take each situation and event to bring you one step closer to achieving your goals. Every moment that passes, you will be closer to your goal.

6. **Meditate**

It's hard to stay focused because daily life tends to distract us with its ups, downs, and a thousand more turns, particularly with the hectic life we currently lead. That is why meditating is so necessary, but do not worry. I'm not going to tell you to sit with your legs crossed on a carpet while listening to chants in a language that you don't understand.

You should always have your priorities in mind to help you remain focused and be more open to messages from the Universe. The more you think about them, the more you like them, the more they are drawn to you, and the more you work with them.

That is why it is recommended to start your everyday routine with certain goals in mind until your day is confused by the news and social networks with the views and negativity of other people .... etcetera, etcetera, etcetera.

In many ways, meditation can be done, and you just need to find a moment alone that you can concentrate on. Meditate when preparing breakfast (just look out for hot things) if cooking relaxes you.

When enjoying your morning coffee, you can also take a few extra minutes in a comfortable chair. Do it early if you like to workout, and use the moment to concentrate on your objectives.

What's more, if you think you don't have enough time for all of the above, you should meditate in the shower, and you're guaranteed to have the moment for yourself at least.

7. **Act intentionally**

For those just beginning to research it, the role of action in the attraction process may become a great source of anxiety and uncertainty.

I believe that there is a tendency to take too literally the teachings of the Law of Attraction. Because we always hear statements like "it is our energy that produces, not behaviour," some will misunderstand it, thinking that literally we don't have to do something.

As much as I want to tell you that you can attract what you want just by wanting it, this is not the case. You must behave consciously.

Think about it, so it's not a matter of enchantment.

If you do not have a single publication, you can not make your blog famous, and you can not make money from home, just by wanting it.

It is not about acting to act now, but about doing it to do what we have chosen to manifest, setting aside preconceived ideas of how exactly it should be.

Most of us humans survive by behaving instinctively (four years ago, including myself). Without really thinking about our every step, we get up, get ready to go to work, and begin our day.

But if you behave deliberately, since they will encourage you and scare you a little at the same time, you will know the sort of acts you can take. You won't always feel relaxed at the beginning, because it means doing something you've never done before, and maybe it will push you out of your comfort zone.

Your mind will have some objections, but you'll know that it's a positive thing and that once you've done it, it will fill you with pride.

8. **Change your environment**

You have to extend this to absolutely everything in life.

You should stay away from lazy people and hang out with businessmen, entrepreneurs, or individuals who aim to be lazy if you want to make more money or start a profitable business.

I recognise that it would be a little harder to change because many do not know that they are the ones who deliberately continue to stay in a toxic environment, and they stagnate because of this.

It will benefit you a great deal to actually change the way you think. Think that there is always a way out of there and start searching for it instead of moaning all day repeating that you can't get out of where you are and that your life will never change.

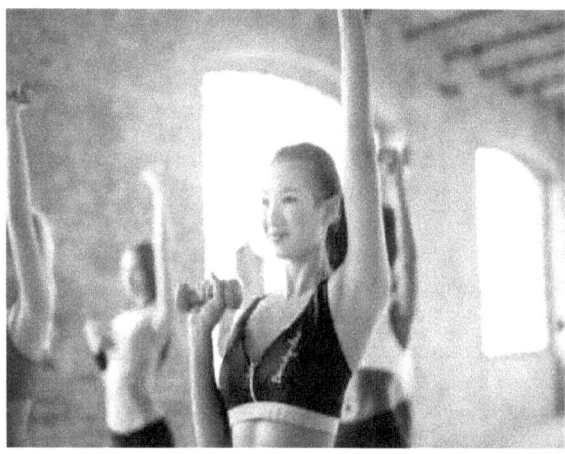

The first step to changing your life is changing your values.

But I didn't even pay attention to those who approached me telling me that I had gone insane when I started writing, thanks to the later shift in my way of looking at things and making one of the best decisions of my life.

Open your mind and let the world and your subconscious find the answers to your problems.

Just as trapped as you believe yourself to be, you are. Take a hard look at your surroundings (things, people, circumstances, career, etc.) and see those that stop you from achieving your goals.

With their negative views and thoughts, maybe some friends or family are keeping you back, or maybe your house is still dirty, and that doesn't encourage you to concentrate. It may also happen that you are exhausted too much by the job you are actually doing, to the extent that you feel that you have no room for anything else.

Through this appraisal, it is imperative that you be truthful and then continue to make the required improvements in your community. I promise you that you will notice a major change in your life if you do.

Only when you go beyond visualizing and daydreaming does the Law of Attraction work. Your mind and HANDS must be put to work simultaneously.

Tools That Will Help You Properly Apply the Law of Attraction

- **Vision board**

This is a (digital or physical) board / poster with pictures illustrating some of the items that you want to accomplish. From magazines, you can cut out images, google them, or draw and paint them. Do your eyes something fun and simple, use shades of colours you like, and pictures that are striking for you.

The most significant thing is that you put it in a position where every day you can see it. Stick it or use it as a wallpaper on the ceiling of your home, whichever is more open to you. The principle is to look at your board every day and get your emotions evoked in you.

In the Law of Attraction, feelings are strong instruments: the more often you can sense and imagine the things that you want to accomplish, the better.

- **Route map**

Basically, a "route map" is what the name implies. Imagine a game map in which, before achieving the target, you have to go through various levels. If you settle on a job you want and enable it, you can't earn the amount of money you want.

Take the time to write or think about the improvements you need to make (from minor to major) to help you achieve your final objective, and then build the map in the style that you like best.

- **Diary**

Nothing will help you concentrate and etch a target in your mind better than writing about it every morning when you wake up and every night before you go to bed. Just as taking notes enables us to revisit a subject, taking a diary will enable you to document all your goals in your mind.

Many psychologists suggest that if you write about the difficulties that happened during the day before going to sleep, as you sleep, your subconscious can seek to find ways to fix those problems, to achieve your objectives.

And I'm telling you that, after a while, it's also very interesting to read your diary and see how far you have improved.

- **Keep your vibes high**

To keep your vibrations high, you must work on the two main components of your "vibrations": your thoughts and emotions.

Think about those things that make you feel optimistic. That makes you feel happy. That makes you focus on the good things in life. Stay positive and grateful.

Whatever you do, do it from abundance, not from scarcity. Worry about taking care of the information with which you feed your mind. In the previous steps, you will already be acting with discipline and focusing on your goals.

However, even those actions that require some effort, you must do it while maintaining optimism and trying to enjoy the process.

Also, make sure that every day you do at least one action that fills you with joy. Try to generate as many positive feelings as possible, and you will be ready to finish the last step and start attracting.

Find as many moments when you feel good and try to make the most of them. Be aware of that joy and enthusiasm, and thus you will be emitting positive frequencies that the Law of Attraction will translate into benefits for you.

Surround yourself with happy people and a positive environment. You will have more energy. The rest will only be to receive and cultivate the results of all the previous steps from now on.

It sounds nice, but how do I know this is effective?

Next, I will share with you why I believe that all this is not simply something abstract and esoteric, as many believe and that it can be very effective if you apply the mentioned steps. To do this, let's analyze some of the elements that make the previous seven steps so effective:

- **High vibrations, better results**

You may be wondering why keeping my vibes high should work? One possible reason is that you will immediately begin to feel better and experience positive emotions by exchanging your negative thoughts for positive ones.

In turn, your positive emotions will cause your mood to change, and as a consequence, you begin to take more actions aligned with your desires.

And as you can imagine, the more actions consistent with the goals you take, the better results you will begin to obtain.

Positive Thoughts →

Positive Emotions →

Positive Actions →

_____

= Positive Results

Thoughts → Emotions → Actions = Results

- **Focus on objectives**

According to various studies, the simple fact of setting goals and objectives increases your chances of achieving the proposed objectives by around 50%. This is precisely where the importance of the Law of Attraction lies.

Defining clearly what you want and setting yourself clear objectives is ALWAYS the first step to achieving them, because how on earth are you going to achieve something that you have not defined? Yes, you may achieve this by chance, but if you leave everything to chance, your odds are against it.

- **Coincidences welcome**

As we mentioned, it is possible that when you begin to apply "the secret," mysteriously, the opportunities begin to appear as if by magic and that the coincidences happen in your favor. But there is an explanation for them. It is the famous RAS.

The RAS, which represents Reticular System Articulation, is responsible for many of these coincidences and opportunities.

The RAS is responsible for our brain filtering and discarding certain information that it does not consider useful for us. It focuses mainly on what it identifies as important.

And it is precisely by clearly defining our wishes and setting specific objectives that we put the RAS to work in our favor.

This is the reason why when we buy a car or car of a certain brand, we begin to come across the same model everywhere that we did not notice before.

The RAS works as a filter that pays attention only to your goals, what you determined is important to you, and all the events, people, or opportunities relevant to your goals.

As you can see, the beginning of achieving what you want is to identify and define it.

When you have done it, you will begin to see more and more opportunities, coincidences, and even "miracles" (identified by the RAS) that may have happened before our noses. Still, because we are not focused enough on it, we probably have not seen it.

- **Successful interactions**

As social beings that we are, many of the goals we set for ourselves depend on collaboration and interaction with other people. But is collaboration and interaction with other people related to the Law of Attraction?

If we consider that those people who apply this law are determined, optimistic, cheerful, and enthusiastic, it is not surprising that they produce good emotions in others. All this generates much more successful interpersonal relationships, which in many cases cause synergies, the collaboration of others, and many opportunities that these people did not obtain before behaving like this.

Few people like to share, tell about an interesting project, or create close bonds with negative, un-optimistic, and low-energy individuals. This increase in your degree of influence on others is one more reason that can positively tilt the balance towards the achievement of your goals if you apply the "The Secret."

- **Increase in key skills**

As if that were not enough, it is no secret that people who keep their vibrations high and report feeling happier tend to considerably increase their performance.

This increase in positive emotions is accompanied by an increase in people's creativity and directs their focus towards solutions instead of problems and increases their productivity and efficiency.

All of this translates into even greater results.

- **Favorable interpretations**

If you consider previous steps, which postulate that you must have absolute faith and take every situation that comes your way as something that will bring you one step closer to your goal, that mentality will likely bear fruit.

Suppose you interpret everything that happens to you as something positive. In that case, mentality-oriented to get the best out of each situation likely leads you to find opportunities where others only see limitations.

It's not so much about what cards you get handed, but how you play them and what you do with them.

- **The more actions you take, the luckier you will have**

As we saw in step number 4, constantly taking action and giving your best effort every day will allow you to access a new world of possibilities.

The more actions you take, the more skills you are constantly acquiring, and the more knowledge you gather, the more capable you will be by the time a great opportunity presents itself by mere coincidence and "luck":

However, it will not be luck. You can take advantage of that opportunity EXCLUSIVELY because you have worked to be prepared for that moment when it comes your way.

That opportunity, it becomes such, the moment you are up to it. Otherwise, it would be something you would not be prepared for and would immediately rule it out.

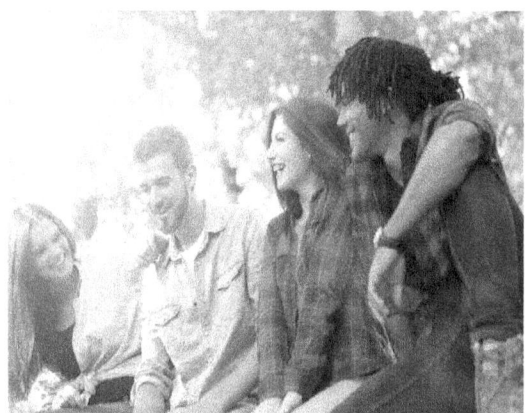

As they say, two phrases that I like a lot:

1. The more I work, the luckier I have
2. The "luck" is the preparation for meeting the opportunity.

Like time, it takes work and preparation. Remember that the most important thing about this law is its last letters:

Law of ATTR-ACTION.

- **Universe factor**

If you still have doubts regarding the effectiveness of this, we can still consider what we will call the "universe" factor.

The Law of Attraction postulates that the Universe gives us back what we focus on. If our energy (thoughts, feelings, and beliefs) is in harmony and aligned with our desires, then the Universe will give us what is necessary to meet these.

"Everything that we think and feel for a long time is what we attract." That is why we must feel as if what we want to happen has already happened. If we do so, the universe will operate as a mirror that will reflect it and send it back to us in the form of situations, events, people, opportunities, or coincidences.

Some call it *synchronicity*: every person encounters events that are in sync with their same frequency.

What do you think?

Regardless of our position on the matter, we must admit that no matter how wise we think we are, we know very little about the Universe.

Although certain physics laws have allowed great advances and a much greater understanding of everything that surrounds us, the truth is that we know little and nothing about the Universe's operation.

Currently, it has been found that 99% of the atoms are composed of VACUUM. We have no idea what everything around us is made of in its smallest degree!

Given the big picture and admitting that we don't know enough, we have two options:

- Believe that the Universe acts in our favor if we follow these steps.
- Believe that the Universe has no interest in us and does not act for or against us regardless of what we do.

When in doubt, I choose option number 1.

"If you want to find the secrets of the universe, think in terms of energy, frequency, and vibration" – is what Nikola Tesla himself said.

This technique is about continuous reflection, being attentive to everything that goes through the mind. Most thoughts are connected to events in the past. To which we go around and around, without reaching anything productive.

Homestretch

May the past help you to learn and know how to act in similar situations. But it makes no sense to keep thinking about something that has already happened, and you cannot change. It is a waste of energy in your life.

Nor is it fruitful to think about the future all the time. It's okay to visualize what you want, plan some actions to achieve your achievements, and connect your energy with that feeling. But everything must be from your today, from the present. Stop hitting the walls.

The past is past, and the future is sometimes uncertain. You must focus on the thoughts that you generate in each moment, to convert them into words and actions that promote the energy necessary for the universe to motorize the frequency and receive the same energy.

The Thought Review Technique may be difficult at first, but I assure you it is worth the reward. You will realize the time and energy you waste on things that will not lead you to achieve your goals.

Sometimes you tend to boycott yourself. With thoughts, feelings, words, and actions that do not correspond to the energy, it takes to produce good things.

Complaining, mocking, being aware of other people's lives will only lead to negativity in your life, which will attract more negativity. So, by constantly checking within your mind, you may find yourself thinking about negative things. It is at that moment when you must raise awareness and change.

You have the power to control and eliminate the negative, replacing it with positive thoughts. In all situations that come your way, you will always have the alternative to opt for a different approach. Highlight the good in people, focus your energy on how to help, and put yourself in the shoes of others.

A very routine example is finding a neighbor who does not say hello. You are in front of your door, and the neighbor passes by and does not say good morning. It is common for your mind to immediately work what a rude neighbor! And there your mind begins to fly but negatively.

Don't say hello to them anymore, cut them off, and discuss it with other neighbors. Now, what you may not know is that that person is going through a bad time. Or you may have a problem, an ailment, or you are simply distracted. And you wasted all that time and energy hooking on something that wasn't real.

On the other hand, the environment and the people around you have an important influence on your life. Stay away from toxic people (even if they are familiar), who are always complaining and charge you with negative energy. Talk to them and change the subject; do not waste time in meaningless discussions and help everyone you can, remember the power of attraction. If you can't find an atmosphere of harmony, you'd better stay away.

Positive thinking will help you overcome fears. And step by step, you will be able to visualize what you want until you begin to decree it, affirm it, and take it into action.

Once your mind is on the positive frequency, and you have begun to visualize what you want for your life, it is time to decree it. The universe will hear your voice, feel the energy of your affirmations, and respond to you. If you are convinced, everything will flow.

You should also complete your thoughts with actions and start executing tasks to make your dreams tangible. It is not just about thinking something and sitting down and waiting for the universe to grant it to you; work for it in your daily life, in the details.

Repeat in your mind and out loud, the affirmations of what you deserve. Go out and look around you, be grateful for what surrounds you, give whoever needs it a look, a smile, a warm word, or a hug; I assure you that it will make a difference.

On a final note, I would like to thank all the people involved mentally, physically, and emotionally in helping me jot down these chapters every night. Thanks to coffee for existing and Oscar, my sweet doggo, putting up with me these weeks.

Wear your mask, my friends. And wash your hands.

Finally, if you enjoyed this book, please let me know your thoughts with a short review on Amazon. All that you need to do is to click the blue link next to the yellow stars that says "customer reviews." You'll then see a gray button that says "Write a customer review"—click that and you're good to go. It means a lot, thank you!

Caryl

Copyright 2020

All Rights Reserved. No part of this book may be reproduced in any form without permission in writing from the author. Reviewers may quote brief passages in reviews.

Disclaimer: No part of this publication may be reproduced or transmitted in any form or by any means, mechanical or electronic, including photocopying or recording, or by any information storage and retrieval system, or transmitted by email without permission in writing from the publisher.

While all attempts have been made to verify the information provided in this publication, neither the author nor the publisher assumes any responsibility for errors, omissions, contrary interpretations of the subject matter herein, or liability whatsoever on behalf of the purchaser or reader of these materials.

www.ingramcontent.com/pod-product-compliance
Lightning Source LLC
Chambersburg PA
CBHW050252010526
44107CB00003B/297